T0258790

HEALTH CARE TRANSITION IN URBAN CHINA

Health Care Transition in Urban China

Edited by

GERALD BLOOM
Institute of Development Studies, Sussex, UK

SHENGLAN TANG
Liverpool School of Tropical Medicine, UK

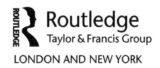

Routledge
Taylor & Francis Group

LONDON AND NEW YORK

First published 2004 by Ashgate Publishing

Published 2016 by Routledge
2 Park Square, Milton Park, Abingdon, Oxon OX14 4RN
711 Third Avenue, New York, NY 10017, USA

Routledge is an imprint of the Taylor & Francis Group, an informa business

British Library Cataloguing in Publication Data
Health care transition in urban china
    1. Medical care - China 2. Health care reform - China 3. Urban
    health - China 4. Sociology, Urban - China
    I. Bloom, Gerald II. Tang, Sheng-lan
    362.1'0951

Library of Congress Cataloging-in-Publication Data
Health care transition in urban china / edited by Gerald Bloom and Shenglan Tang.
    p. cm.
    Includes bibliographical references and index.
    ISBN 978-0-7546-3966-4
    1. Health care reform--China. 2. Urban health--China. 3. Health services
accessibility--China. 4. Medical care--China. I. Bloom, Gerald. II. Shenglan, Tang,
1962-

    RA395.C53H436 2004
    362.1'0425'0951--dc22

                                 2004052482
ISBN 9780754639664 (hbk)

Transfered to Digital Printing in 2010

Contents

List of Figures

List of Tables

List of Boxes

List of Contributors

Ying Bian is a Senior Lecturer at the Centre for Health Management and Policy at Shandong University. He gained his MPH and Ph.D. from Shandong Medical University. His research interests are hospital costing, regional health planning and health policy studies. He has conducted a number of research projects with grants from the World Health Organization and China's Ministry of Health and published a number of research articles.

Gerald Bloom is the leader of the Health and Social Change Team at the Institute of Development Studies at the University of Sussex, UK. He is a medical doctor and economist with expertise in health policy, planning and finance in low- and middle-income countries. He has participated in studies of a number of aspects of health sector reform in China. He has also provided technical support to several Chinese government health reform and development initiatives. He is Deputy Chairman of the China Health Development Forum.

Jiaying Chen works in Nanjing Medical University as Director of the Department of Health Policy and Management. He is also Vice-President of Jiangsu Provincial Society of Health Economics. Dr Chen is involved in the Jiangsu Health Modernization project and is working in the field of health system development, especially the privatization of township health centres and cooperative medical schemes.

Youlong Gong is Professor of the Department of Health Statistics and Social Medicine, School of Public Health, Fudan University. He is chairperson of the Chinese Association of Social Medicine. His professional activities focus on health services research and health human resource planning and projection. He is currently involved in projects on TB control and social assessment, and shigellosis vaccine acceptance assessment.

Yuelai Lu is a Senior Research Associate in the Overseas Development Group at the University of East Anglia, UK, and Executive Secretary of the China Health Development Forum at the Institute of Development Studies at the University of Sussex, UK.

Henry Lucas is a Fellow of the Institute of Development Studies at the University of Sussex, UK. He is a statistician who has specialized in information systems, monitoring and evaluation and research methods. He has worked for many years on health sector analysis and more recently on the monitoring of Poverty Reduction Strategies. He has been principal researcher in a number of recent studies involving the combination of quantitative and qualitative/participatory fieldwork methods. These have included: a review of the Malawi Social Action Fund; an exploration of the links between energy, poverty and gender in poor rural areas of China; and monitoring a Department for International Development health care programme in Nigeria. He has more than ten years of research and consultancy experience on both rural and urban health care in China.

Qingyue Meng is a Professor in Health Economics and directs the Centre for Health Management and Policy at Shandong University. He has an MD from Shandong Medical University, an MPH from Shanghai Medical University and an MA from the School of Economics of the University of the Philippines. He is currently a member of the advisory committee on health policy and management to China's Ministry of Health. He has conducted a number of research projects with grants from the World Bank, World Health Organization, UNICEF and domestic funding agencies. His research interests include health care financing, hospital costing and pricing policy and economic evaluation of health programmes. He has published two books and numerous research articles.

Xu Qian is currently Professor and Director of the Department of Maternal and Child Health at Fudan University School of Public Health. She also serves as Deputy Dean of the School of Public Health and Vice-President of the Chinese Maternal Health Care Association. Since 1990 Dr Qian has undertaken a number of research projects including evaluating and supervising the China–UNICEF MCH/FP projects for ten years and advising on and monitoring the Ningxia MCH/FP project supported by AusAid.

Clas Rehnberg is Associate Professor in Health Economics, Medical Management Centre, Karolinska Institutet, Stockholm, Sweden. His research interests are the reform of health systems and health care financing and delivery. Currently he is engaged in studies of the regulation of the pharmaceutical sector in low- and middle-income countries. He has been a consultant for the World Bank, World Health Organization, the European Commission and other international institutions. He has many years' teaching experience in health economics and health policy including management programmes for executives and senior physicians.

Baogang Shu is Professor of the Department of Health Statistics and Social Medicine, School of Public Health, Fudan University. His professional activities focus on health statistics, especially multiple regression analysis. He is involved in projects on health care reform and MCH in poor rural areas of China.

Hilary Standing is a Fellow of the Institute of Development Studies at the University of Sussex, UK. She is a social anthropologist specializing in health research and social development. Current interests include: household-level and gender aspects of health and formal and informal care systems; gender and equity in the context of health reforms; the management of organizational change in health sector restructuring, especially the changing roles of providers; and improving accountability within health systems. She has worked extensively in rural and urban South Asia and convenes the international Gender and Health Equity Network.

Qiang Sun MD, MPH is a Lecturer at the Centre for Health Management and Policy, Shandong University. His research fields include the assessment of health sector reform, drug pricing and the impact of economic globalization on the health system.

Shenglan Tang is Senior Lecturer in International Health at the Liverpool School of Tropical Medicine, UK. His research experience is in the areas of health policy, health systems development and disease control with special reference to equity and efficiency.

Rachel Tolhurst is a Research Associate and Doctoral Candidate at the Liverpool School of Tropical Medicine (LSTM). She has an MA in Gender and Development and has developed Guidelines for the Analysis of Gender and Health with the Gender and Health Group at LSTM. Her research interests are in gender and equity in relation to health systems development and communicable disease, and qualitative and participatory research in health. She has studied Chinese language at degree level and has been involved in several qualitative research projects in China.

Thomas Uhlemann is a social scientist/sociologist, specializing in medical sociology and international comparison of health care systems. He conducted studies in sociology, history and political science at the University of Göttingen, 1983–92. He worked in social research in medical sociology at the University of Göttingen, 1992–2001 and was Assistant Professor at the Institute of Medical Sociology, Medical School, University of Hamburg. Since 2002 Dr Uhlemann has been Research Fellow at the AOK Research Institute, Bonn (AOK is the largest health insurance company in Germany). His current research interests include health care systems, public health, social impact of economic reforms and transition and illness behaviour.

Wei Wang is Assistant Professor in the Department of Health Statistics and Social Medicine, School of Public Health, Fudan University. Dr Wang is now participating in the Operation of Community Health Services in four Urban Health and Poverty Project cities in China. She is also involved in the Qualitative Study for Urban Health Reform as part of the Third National Health Survey and the Social Assessment of TB Control Project in China.

Zhonghua Weng is Associate Professor of the Department of Health Statistics and Social Medicine, School of Public Health, Fudan University. She has worked on data analysis and computer techniques and is now involved in projects on TB social economic evaluation and shigellosis vaccine acceptance assessment.

Fei Yan is Associate Professor and Vice-Chairperson of the Department of Health Statistics and Social Medicine, School of Public Health, Fudan University and a committee member of the Shanghai Association of Social Medicine. She is now involved in the Urban Health and Poverty Project and working on the Operation of Community Health Services in four project cities in China. She is also involved in the project of Qualitative Study for Urban Health Reform as part of the Third National Health Survey. In addition, Dr Yan acts as national consultant on the Social Assessment of TB Control Project in China.

Ning Zhuang is a Programme Officer in the Department of Health Planning and Finance of the Ministry of Health, China. He received his MD and MPH from Shandong Medical University where he was involved in the European Union–China urban health project. His current responsibility in the Ministry of Health includes the development of health care and drug pricing policy.

Acknowledgements

This book reports the findings of a research project undertaken by three Chinese and three European institutions: the School of Public Health of Fudan University, the Institute of Social Medicine and Health Policy of Shandong University, the Chinese Health Economics Institute (which replaced the former Department of Health Policy and Law of the Ministry of Health), the Institute of Development Studies (IDS), UK, Stockholm School of Economics, Sweden, and the Institute of Medical Sociology of the University of Hamburg, Germany. Dr Shenglan Tang, of Fudan University/Liverpool School of Tropical Medicine, was Scientific Coordinator and Dr Gerald Bloom, of the IDS, was Administrative Coordinator.

This project was supported by a grant from the Research Directorate-General of the European Commission (Contract No. IC18CT980343). The Department for International Development (DFID) of the British Government co-funded the equity study. The Ford Foundation provided a small grant to Professor Xu Qian and Ms Rachel Tolhurst from Fudan University and the Liverpool School of Tropical Medicine for a gender analysis study of access to health care. During the final editing of the book, Gerald Bloom was a Distinguished Associate Fellow of the Institute for Advanced Study of LaTrobe University, Melbourne, Australia.

The UK DFID supports policies, programmes and projects to promote international development. DFID provided funds for this study as part of that objective but the views and opinions expressed are those of the authors alone. The same disclaimer applies to the European Commission and the Ford Foundation.

The project received support from a number of institutions and individuals in China and Europe. A number of government departments in Jiangsu and Shandong Provinces and in Nantong and Zibo Municipalities provided important assistance. The Medical Insurance Management Centre in Nantong and the Municipal Health Bureaux in the two cities were particularly helpful. We would like to thank particularly the following people for their kind assistance: Huang Deming, Miao Baoying, Cao Jinhai, Lu Huijun and Zhang Bing from Nantong, and Zhao Yicheng, Zhang Xixun, Li Wei, and Zhao Yanfeng from Zibo.

Our sincere thanks are due to the following individuals who provided support throughout the project: Dr Anna Karaoglou of the European Commission in Brussels, Dr Joan Kaufman, then Programme Officer of Ford Foundation, Dr Minghui Ren, Deputy Director-General of the Department of International Cooperation of the Ministry of Health, Beijing, and Professor Qingwu Jiang, Dean of the School of Public Health of Fudan University. We would also like to thank Sarah Cook, Joan Kaufman and James Killingsworth for providing very helpful comments on chapters of the draft research report during the Beijing Conference. Karen Ross-Millianos, a research assistant from the IDS, made great efforts to edit each chapter of the original research report, for which the researchers of the project were very grateful.

List of Abbreviations

ACWF	All China Women's Federation
AES	Anti-Epidemic Station
CASS	Chinese Academy of Social Sciences
CDC	Centre for Disease Control and Prevention
CHSI	Centre for Health Statistics and Information
CMI	case mix index
CMS	Cooperative Medical System
COE	collectively owned enterprise
DEA	data envelopment analysis
DFID	Department for International Development
DRG	diagnosis related group
GIS	Government Insurance Scheme
HIS	Health Insurance Scheme
ILO	International Labour Organization
LIS	Labour Insurance Scheme
LOS	length of stay
MCH	maternal and child health
MLS	minimum living security
MMR	maternal mortality rate
MOH	Ministry of Health
MOLSS	Ministry of Labour and Social Security
NCD	non-communicable disease
NHSS	National Health Services Survey
PHC	primary health care
PL	poverty line
QAI	quality adjusted index
SARS	Severe Acute Respiratory Syndrome
SOE	state-owned enterprise
SPSS	Statistical Package for the Social Sciences
STD	sexually transmitted disease
THC	township health centre
U5MR	under-five mortality rate
UNDP	United Nations Development Programme
WHO	World Health Organization

Foreword

It is a great pleasure to write a foreword for this important and useful publication. As part of its overall research programme, the European Commission provides substantial funds every year for research into health and development. The overriding objective is to increase knowledge that can be used to enhance the health of the poor. This document is the product of one such research project and is intended to strengthen an area which is of increasing importance – improving equity and efficiency of the urban health services with the aim of 'making research count'.

Whilst considerable knowledge exists on the causes of ill-health and technical interventions that could improve the levels of health, there is far less understanding as to how such interventions should be implemented. Some of the problems encountered are undoubtedly attributable to poor planning systems. This report, which stems from collaborative research between European and Chinese partner institutions, provides useful and accessible guidance for planners as to how to link research to health system development and the importance of strengthening the links with policy-makers within the context of a research project. The EC is proud to have supported such research as a contribution to the enhancement of community health services as well as a contribution to the needs of the poorest.

Dr Anna Karaoglou,
European Commission, DG Research,
International Scientific Cooperation

Introduction

China has been in transition to a market economy since the late 1970s. The changes under way are having a profound impact on almost every aspect of urban health services, and there has been a growing recognition by the general public and decision-makers of the need for urban health system reform. The government has acknowledged the importance of this issue in a series of policy statements, making health one of the key areas of concern in the current stage of transition.

This study, developed in consultation with the Ministry of Health, sought systematic evidence of the effect of changes in health finance on the performance of urban health services in terms of equity and efficiency, as well as of the impact of certain reform initiatives. The project took the form of comparative case studies in Nantong, Jiangsu Province, and Zibo, Shandong Province. It was anticipated that this approach would generate an in-depth understanding of the relationship between transition, health reform and health system performance in medium-sized cities. One reason for the choice of the two cities is that their governments have actively supported innovative approaches to health system development.

An important area that came to the fore during research was the relationship between the shifting socio-economic environment – particularly the changing pattern of urban employment and attendant benefit entitlements due to enterprise reform – and access to health services. It became clear that a growing proportion of the urban population is not eligible for employment-related health benefits or is only entitled to reduced benefits, and, depending on profit levels, even these may not be paid. Moreover, in the shift to a market economy, many have been marginalized and impoverished, making it harder for them to afford rising out-of-pocket health expenses. Although such inequity might be expected in such a transition, China has particular problems due to her past emphasis on a publicly owned economic system.

Whilst the urban population has mushroomed in the last two decades, enterprise reform, particularly since the mid-1990s, has led to an increasing number of bankrupt enterprises and job cuts, especially in the state-owned sector. In 1980 most enterprise employees worked for state-owned or collectively owned enterprises; by 2000 these categories accounted for only about half of enterprise employees. For many urban employees, permanent employment contracts have given way to fixed-term contracts or temporary jobs. These changes have had a major impact on urban health insurance, especially since, in the present system, benefit levels are dependent on the nature of the enterprise and the status of employment. Government officials and business sector managers are particularly concerned about the impact of enterprise reform on the financing of health services for the rising numbers of unemployed and laid-off. Presently, no health insurance protection is available for a large proportion of the unemployed or for the so-called 'floating' population of rural-to-urban migrants. Women in particular suffer from reduced benefit coverage since they are over-represented in groups which have short-term contracts or are laid off.

To compound the situation, health care costs have escalated. In 1999 10.5 per cent of government expenditure was allocated to health in Nantong, contributing to just over 14 per cent of total health expenditure. Hospitals raise additional revenue through user charges. In 1997 drug sales accounted for 50 per cent of hospital income in municipal and county hospitals in Zibo. The high cost of health care and spotty insurance coverage have prompted concerns about the access to medical services of vulnerable groups such as the elderly, indigent, disabled and migrants, whose numbers are increasing. In 1998 it was estimated that approximately 44 per cent of China's city-dwellers were uninsured.

Faced with no health insurance, or an employer which is unable to afford reimbursements, people ration treatment and medicines, frequently only seeking help when an illness becomes serious. Sadly, the vulnerable, especially the poor, have been hardest hit. For some households, an incidence of chronic ill-health is likely to propel the family into complete destitution. Moreover, all of this is occurring in the context of demographic transition to an ageing society, and one in which the epidemiological profile has shifted from communicable to non-communicable diseases, producing an increasing prevalence rate of chronic illness. This study clearly points to the need for investment in public health education and preventive programmes. It also highlights the need for development of indicators of vulnerability in tandem with additional state programmes for the coverage of health costs, especially for the poor. Developing basic, affordable community health services would also increase the availability and accessibility of health care for the vulnerable.

In addition to the issue of equity in access to health services, various factors negatively affecting the efficiency of the public health system have drawn attention to the necessity for reform. In addition to costly and excessive prescription of medicines, which we have noted, other factors include irrational allocation of health resources and poor staff management. A number of hospital-related reforms have been initiated since the 1980s concentrating on hospital reimbursement mechanisms, price controls, health insurance reform, payment methods and regional health planning. However, entrenched problems persist and more needs to be done.

The chief factors impacting negatively on efficiency mainly stem from the way the health system is financed. The system of allocation of government health budgets on the basis of the numbers of beds and staff has had some influence. Pressure to generate revenue has led health workers to encourage the use of expensive technologies and over-prescribe drugs. Incentives for such practices include bonuses paid by hospitals to individual personnel or departments which, since 1994, have been allocated according to measures of performance, the most important being revenue generation. The average costs of out-patient and in-patient visits increased rapidly in both cities in the 1990s, while utilization of these services declined. The latter can be attributed to not only medical care costs, but also the reduction in coverage of employment-related health insurance, and increasing competition. At the same time, whilst activity per health worker and per bed fell, income per health worker rose in both cities during the 1990s. With regard to personnel policy, although this has been reformed according to government guidelines and health workers now work on contracts, hospital managers still experience pressure to appoint recommended people, and find it difficult to fire staff. Hence, hospitals are experiencing declining productivity and low utilization of services, coupled with expansion of hospitals in size, staff and investment in high-tech equipment.

Attempts at reforming municipal health insurance aimed at establishing a general health insurance for all urban residents, and controlling supply and demand, have been implemented since the early 1990s in the form of model projects. In early 1999, a finalized nationwide health care reform plan was launched, which introduced a new Basic Health Insurance Scheme, aimed at eventually superseding the Government Insurance Scheme and the Labour Insurance Scheme. Nantong is one of a relatively small number of cities piloting the new insurance schemes.

Clearly, as the government asserts, it is imperative that comprehensive urban health reforms are devised and implemented. It is hoped that the study presented in this volume will contribute to the design of a new, more equitable, efficient and accessible health system.

One important point that must be stressed is that the milieu in which the study took place is very complex and continually changing. Researchers attempted to gather data and perform analysis in a period of incredibly rapid economic growth and urbanization, when population patterns were (and are) shifting significantly, and health care costs were escalating. In addition, there have been multiple, small-scale urban health reform initiatives, that is continuous reforms, addressing problems as they arose. Consequently, it is impossible to measure the impact of any one.

On top of this, the government's transition strategy is to separate rural and urban. As a result, we are not dealing with a single geographically based system. Zibo, for example, has five scattered satellite areas which constitute the urban area, and statistically Nantong is frequently delineated into Nantong Municipality, composed of all urban and rural areas, and 'downtown Nantong'. Moreover, the boundary between rural and urban changes as urbanization proceeds, making it exceedingly difficult to isolate trends and, more importantly, calling into question the quality of the data produced (this is indicated in the study where it is obvious). Finally, there is also the issue of the 'registered' population, what we are referring to when the 'population' of the study cities is discussed, and the large 'unregistered' or 'floating' population: migrant workers from rural areas of the province or from outside the province whose numbers are uncertain.

Given all of the above, it is, understandably, tempting to query the significance of the present research study and its findings. What was the rationale one might ask; what exactly were researchers trying to achieve? The answer is that the study has attempted to understand at *one point in time* what the reality is, what the problems are, and what are the potential solutions. The project sought to reveal what is actually happening on the ground in two sample cities, identify the trends and issues and discover how the system is responding. The importance of the study, then, lies in the fact that it provides a snapshot of reality, crystallizing valuable evidence regarding the factors affecting current health system performance at one juncture, which will be of real use to health system planners in devising future reform and development strategies. Obviously, for the reasons stated it has not been easy to capture reality – is it ever? – but we believe the in-depth, wide-ranging quantitative analysis supplemented by numerous histories of individual cases reveals the minutiae of the situation during the study period (1997–2000). The fact that the research team worked closely with policy-makers and local health managers throughout the project to ensure that the study focused on the issues potential users of the findings considered important also bodes well and should guarantee the relevance of the subject matter.

The study is structured as follows. Chapter 1 sets the problems arising with urban health services in the context of a number of simultaneous transitions taking place (economic, demographic, epidemiological) and provides a conceptual framework for assessing the performance of local health systems. Chapter 2 provides a review of the recent history of reform initiatives allowing the reader to contextualize the experiences of the two study cities. Chapters 3 and 4 introduce the two study cities, their health problems and the organization of their health systems. Chapters 5, 6, 7 and 8 report on different aspects of the study of access to health services. Chapters 9 and 10 present the findings of the study of the efficiency of hospital services. Chapter 11 presents the conclusions and policy recommendations.

Chapter 1

China in Transition: Challenges to Urban Health Services

Gerald Bloom

China is undergoing a number of simultaneous changes. It is in transition to a market economy and an urbanized and industrialized society. It is rapidly expanding communications within the country and with the rest of the world. Its age structure and patterns of ill-health are also changing. The rapid economic growth has been uneven and this has led to new patterns of social segmentation. This chapter introduces the reader to this dynamic reality and sets the stage for the detailed discussion of the experiences of Nantong and Zibo, two medium-sized cities.

Urbanization

According to official statistics, China is still a largely rural society. However, over the past 20 years the proportion categorized as urban has grown sharply (Table 1.1). In the year 2000, 458 million people were registered as permanent residents of urban areas, or 36.2 per cent of the total population.

Table 1.1 Trends in urban population, 1980–2000

Year	Total population (million)	Urban population (million)	Proportion (%)
1980	987	191	19.4
1985	1,059	251	23.7
1990	1,143	302	26.4
1995	1,211	352	29.0
2000	1,266	458	36.2

Source: China Statistical Yearbook (2001).

In 1980 there were 223 cities, of which 15 had more than a million people (Table 1.2). Twenty years later there were 663 cities, of which 41 were bigger than a million. These changes are due to a combination of in-migration and the reclassification of areas from rural to urban. China classifies cities in terms of their level of administrative autonomy. The governments of Beijing, Tianjin, Shanghai and Chongqing have the same status as provinces. There are 259 cities with prefecture status, the administrative level below the provinces. There are 400 cities with county status.

Table 1.2 Number of cities by size of non-agricultural population

City size	1980	1991	2000
2 million +	7	9	14
1–2 million	8	22	27
0.5–1.0 million	30	30	53
0.2–0.5 million	72	121	218
less than 0.2 million	106	297	352
Total	223	479	663

Source: Song and Zhang (2002) Table 2; *China Statistical Yearbook* (2001).

One cannot simply equate the size of the urban population with the number of people living in cities. The estimates of urban population are based on the registration of individual households as agricultural or non-agricultural. Many non-agricultural households live in small towns in rural counties. On the other hand, most city administrations include localities classified as rural. Many municipalities contain more households with rural registration than urban. This makes interpretation of statistics difficult. It also hints at the difficulties that city governments face in developing population-based social policies.

The numbers in Table 1.1 underestimate the degree of urbanization in China. According to Hussain (1999), 53.4 per cent of the labour force worked in services and industry in the late 1990s and 51 per cent of the population lived in urban settlements, with high population density and a preponderant share of non-farming activities in the local economy. This is much higher that the official figure of 36.2 per cent of people with non-agricultural registration. There are two reasons for this discrepancy. First, the economy of many localities near urban centres is no longer based on agriculture, but their administrative status has not changed to take this into account. For example, many of the so-called rural counties around Shanghai largely depend on non-agricultural production. Second, many migrants to cities are not officially registered as permanent residents.

The changing numbers in Table 1.2 reflect the upgrading of county seats to city status and the upgrading of small urban centres to prefecture status by expanding their territories and/or merging two adjacent cities. The administrative changes have not kept up with the actual rate of urbanization. This is partly due to administrative inertia. It may also reflect the outcome of economic pressures. The classification of a locality as urban has important implications for employment, social security and so forth (Song and Zhang, 2002). Political leaders may want the greater status that urban classification brings. However, they have to consider the impact that a change in classification will have on local enterprises by requiring them to provide more social benefits to their employees. There is an incentive for certain kinds of enterprise to locate in rural areas. This may have contributed to the patchwork model of urbanization.

Classification of a household as urban or rural greatly affects its entitlements. This arises from the system of household registration or *hukou*, established in the cities in 1951 and extended to rural areas in 1955. Registration status has important implications for a household's ability to obtain employment and secure social benefits. Officially sanctioned rural-to-urban migration requires a formal *hukou* transfer from agricultural to non-agricultural status. This process is subject to policy restrictions, defining the desired qualifications, and quota controls. The census data refer to those who have the right to permanent residence in urban areas and not to 'temporary' migrants.

Government regulations require everyone moving to a place and remaining for over one month to register with the local police station and obtain a permission card for residence. This requirement aims to monitor the movement of the so-called floating population in the urban areas. However, many people do not adhere to the above registration. All urban areas have a large number of non-registered residents.

The Chinese refer to those living in a locality where they are not registered as the floating population. However, it is difficult to pin down a clear definition of this term or accurately to estimate its size. This paragraph draws heavily on the paper by Goodkind and West (2002). One source of data is the annual survey of population change, which records the number of people residing away from their household registration location for six months or longer. This number rose from 58.4 million in 1996 to 63.8 million in 1999. Another source of data is the Ministry of Public Security, to which the police report. It estimated the floating population at 100 million in 1997 and projected it would rise further. However, this may include people staying away from home for as little as a day. These data illustrate how difficult it is to define what the floating population is and to measure its size.

Economic and Social Change

China has experienced more than 20 years of sustained economic growth. Between 1978 and 2000 the gross domestic product per capita rose from CNY379 to CNY7,078. After correcting for inflation, gross domestic product (GDP) per capita in 2000 was 5.6 times the level in 1978.[1] Economic growth has led to rapid rises in average income. Annual disposable income per capita for urban households rose from CNY343 in 1978 to CNY6,280 in 2000.[2] The level in 2000 was equivalent to 3.8 times that in 1978, at constant prices. The rise in disposable income has been associated with changes in patterns of consumption. There were 163 bicycles, 91 washing machines, 80 refrigerators and 38 cameras per 100 urban households in 2000.

One sign of the pace of change is the increase in the number of colour television sets per 100 households in urban areas from 17.2 to 116.6 between 1985 and 2000. Even the poorest 10 per cent of urban households had 99 sets per 100 households. Television reached 93.7 per cent of China's population in 2000. This provides an indication of the rapid growth in communication that has accompanied economic growth. Many goods and services, including health-related ones, are now advertised on television, radio and in print media. This has influenced popular expectations.

Economic growth has not been distributed evenly. The eastern parts of the country have developed much more quickly than the west. In 2000 GDP per capita ranged from CNY2,662 in Guizhou to CNY22,460 in Beijing.[3] The government is now giving priority to measures aimed at helping lagging areas to catch up.

There are substantial differences in the economic well-being of households within each locality. In 2000 the poorest 10 per cent of urban households had an annual income of CNY2,678 per capita, compared with CNY13,390 for the richest 10 per cent.[4] These substantial inequalities have a number of effects. On the one hand, the patterns of consumption of the richer groups influence overall expectations through demonstration effects and the power of the media. On the other hand, a group of urban poor have emerged in recent years.

The growing inequality is associated with increasing diversity in types of employment (Table 1.3). In 1980 most urban jobs were in state or collectively owned enterprises. In 2000 employment in the first two categories had fallen, but a large number of people worked for privately owned companies and over 20 million people were self-employed.

Table 1.3 Number of employed people in urban areas by type of employer

	1980 (million)	1985 (million)	1990 (million)	1995 (million)	2000 (million)
State-owned	80.2	89.9	103.5	112.6	81.0
Collectively owned	24.3	33.2	35.5	31.5	15.0
Cooperative	–	–	–	–	1.6
Joint ownership	–	0.4	1.0	0.5	0.4
Limited liability	–	–	–	–	6.9
Share-holding	–	–	–	3.2	4.6
Private	–	–	0.6	4.9	12.7
Funding from Hong Kong, Macau, Taiwan	–	–	0.04	2.7	3.1
Foreign investment	–	0.06	0.6	2.4	3.3
Self-employed	0.8	4.5	6.1	15.6	21.4

Source: China Statistical Yearbook (2001), Table 5.4.

The need to address the problems of unprofitable state-owned enterprises has dominated policy development in urban areas. Beginning in the mid-1980s the government introduced the labour contract system to replace the previous guarantees of work until retirement. The government has encouraged a restructuring of enterprises since the early 1990s. Many laid-off workers have maintained nominal employment relations with their original work units, for fear of losing their work-related entitlements. This makes it difficult to quantify the number of unemployed.

The registered unemployment rate in urban areas has been consistently 3.1 per cent since 1997 according to national statistics.[5] This is the number of people registered as unemployed. However, many more are laid-off. These are people who remain formally attached to their employment units and receive an allowance and some benefits. At the end of 2000 there were 8.6 million laid-off employees and 5.95 million registered unemployed (Hussain, 2003). Gu (2003) estimates that real unemployment rates were 6.99 per cent in 1999, taking the number of laid-off persons into account. He points out that a large proportion of these people live in localities that were previously centres of industrial production. Hu (1999) estimates the unemployment rate at 7.9–8.5 per cent in 1998, taking into account unemployment amongst migrant workers.

According to 1998 national statistics, 66.7 per cent of the laid-off workers were above 35 years of age and almost a quarter were above 46 years. Women do not make up a disproportionate share of the total numbers of laid-off, but since they do not make up half of the workforce the unemployment rate of women, related to their total employment, is high.

Li, Chunling (2002) claims that a complex pattern of social segmentation has emerged in the cities over the past decade or so. At the top are those with social influence and/or financial power. Then come a variety of categories of salaried workers, middle-managers and small business owners. At the bottom of the social scale are the urban poor and vulnerable. They include laid-off workers, the unemployed and those who cannot work (Cook, 2001).

The government has defined minimum living standards for urban areas, below which people are entitled to financial support. According to a survey by the Ministry of Civil Affairs, around 14 million urban residents had an income below the local poverty line in 2000. Hussain (2003) points out that it is difficult to interpret the meaning of this figure. First, cities establish their own poverty lines below which benefits are paid. In 2000 they varied from CNY2,400 to CNY3,828 per person in some of the largest cities, from CNY1,680 to CNY2,400 in many of the provincial capitals and even lower in prefecture-level cities. The poverty lines reflect differences in the cost of living and in the capacity of city governments to pay income supplements. Also, poverty lines for residents of 'rural' counties within municipal boundaries are much lower. Many more people have incomes just above the poverty line. This suggests that quite large numbers of people are poor or at risk of impoverishment. This has important implications for social policy.

Demographic Change

The structure of China's population is changing rapidly owing to an active family planning policy and factors associated with economic and social development. Average life expectancy has been rising. Table 1.4 shows the fall in the proportion of the population below the age of 15 years and the rise in the number of elderly. The proportion over 65 years grew from 3.6 per cent in 1964 to 7.0 per cent in 2000. The proportion over 75 years old more than doubled from 0.8 per cent in 1964 to 2.2 per cent in 2000.

The ageing of the population is expected to continue. The China Population Information and Research Centre projects that the percentage over 65 years will rise to 8 per cent by 2010, 11 per cent in 2020 and 20 per cent in 2040. In 1990 around 30 per cent of people over 65 were over 75 years; this proportion is projected to rise to 35 per cent in 2010 and around 50 per cent in 2050 (Sun, 1998).

Table 1.4 Age structure of China from 1964 to 2000

Age	1964 (%)	1982 (%)	1990 (%)	2000 (%)
0–14	40.7	33.6	27.7	22.9
15–64	55.8	61.5	66.7	70.2
65+	3.6	4.9	5.6	7.0
75+	0.8	1.4		2.2

Source: China Statistical Yearbooks (1998; 2001) and CHSI preliminary analysis of 2000 Census.

Changing Patterns of Medical Need

This section explores how these changes are affecting the need for health services. Williams (1991) defines medical need as the existence of ill-health for which an effective treatment is available. The amount of need is a measure of the physiological and psychological status of individuals, their expectations of what constitutes well-being, the availability of effective interventions and the social arrangements that determine the roles of households and health providers in caring for the sick. According to this definition, need is determined by the burden of sickness and the social consensus about the kinds of support sick individuals require. Both determinants are changing.

Demographic change has been associated with an epidemiological transition. The incidence of infectious diseases has fallen dramatically, related to improvements in the standard of living and specific public health measures. The ageing of the population and high rates of risky behaviour, such as smoking, have led to increases in the prevalence of non-communicable diseases. Recent studies amongst the elderly identify a number of problems with chronic disease (Deng *et al.*, 1999; Ou and Zhu, 2000; Zhou and Wang, 1998).

Data from advanced market economies suggest that average medical care costs rise rapidly with age (Barer *et al.*, 1987). Those over 75 years old have a particularly great need for expensive health care. The aged account for a substantial share of medical care costs in urban China. A brief analysis of the disbursements of Shenyang's government insurance scheme by one of the authors indicated large differences in utilization between age groups. Pensioners spent 2.3 times as much as current employees; veterans of the liberation war (many over 75 years old) spent twice as much again. These differences reflect, in part, the special entitlements that these veterans have. They also reflect the high levels of need associated with old age. Pressure on the medical system is likely to grow as the numbers of the elderly increase.

The high cost of care for the elderly also reflects changes to family structures, which have made people less able and willing to care for very dependent people at home (Xiong, 1999). The lack of affordable medical support for the aged puts a heavy burden on family caregivers, particularly women.

Demographic transition affects pensions and health services differently. The rise in the number of pensioners is well advanced. The ratio of pensioners to workers rose from 1:12.8 to 1:4.8 between 1980 and 1995 (West, 1999). This is partly due to the ageing of the population. It is also due to a cohort effect, as the generation who began work during the 1950s reaches retirement age, and to the government policy of encouraging early retirement as a means of reducing open unemployment. The cost of health care continues to increase beyond retirement age and the rise in cost of health insurance is likely to lag 10–15 years behind the rise in pensions. By this reckoning, the need for medical care will continue to rise rapidly over the next few years.

The changing expectations of urban dwellers also influence medical need. Their tastes have been strongly affected by the spread of communications, which has increased their knowledge about lifestyles elsewhere. They have also been affected by the marketing of medical products. These factors have combined to alter the expectations of providers and users of health services. The disposable income of urban dwellers has grown rapidly and health expenditure has grown even faster (Zhao, 1999). The disposable income of the highest social strata has grown faster still. Members of the political elite, such as the veterans of the revolutionary war, are entitled to free treatment at the most sophisticated facilities. These factors have encouraged the development of a costly style of high-technology care.

The locus of care has largely shifted from clinics and simple in-patient facilities to out-patient departments and wards of sophisticated hospitals. The consumption of drugs, particularly expensive branded products, has grown rapidly. In 1993, 52 per cent of total health expenditure in China was on pharmaceuticals (World Bank, 1997). Expenditure on other inputs has also risen rapidly. The Ministry of Health (1998a) recently reported that 50 per cent of 3,640 county and higher level hospitals had a computed axial tomography (CT) scanner. This reflects the proliferation of diagnostic and treatment technologies.

The shift towards a more expensive style of medical care reflects the availability of expensive, but effective, interventions and a growth in demand for them. It also reflects cost increases related to government policies. Government health budgets have risen less rapidly than salary costs. Despite this, some local governments have encouraged health facilities to employ more staff. Health facilities have had to generate revenue to meet the income expectations of their employees (Bloom *et al.*, 2000). The government has controlled the price of a consultation with a health worker and a day in hospital, whilst allowing health facilities to earn a mark-up on drug sales and the use of sophisticated equipment. This has encouraged costly forms of practice (Wu, 2002). During the early 1980s, when new patterns of service provision were being established, there were few pensioners over 75 years of age and enterprises could afford sophisticated hospital care. By the 1990s an expensive style of care had become the norm. Recent government policy statements seek to reverse this trend through a number of measures to control hospital costs and by encouraging cities to establish community health centres as an alternative to hospital out-patient departments (see Chapter 2).

Recent surveys have found that urban residents are becoming increasingly concerned about the high cost of medical care. A survey conducted by the Chinese Statistical Bureau at the end of 2000 found that 87 per cent of respondents identified the high cost of medical care as their most serious concern (Gong, 2001).

At the other end of the spectrum are the poor and vulnerable. There is little systematic information on their living conditions and health situation. There are indications that they have more health problems and less access to services than other city dwellers. Some studies link psychological problems to the experience of being laid off (Zhang *et al.*, 1999; Chen and Guo, 2000). Several studies of rural-to-urban migrants have reported higher incidence of infectious diseases. Chen (2000) associates the resurgence of tuberculosis and sexually transmitted diseases (STDs) in the cities with rapid urbanization. Wang *et al.* (2000) report that 60 per cent of cases of STD were associated with migrants in Xiaoshan City, Zhejiang.

Two recent surveys show that urban residents are experiencing increasing difficulty in gaining access to health services (Gao *et al.*, 2001). In 1992 20 per cent of people referred to hospital declined admission and 40 per cent of them said it was due to cost; five years later 32 per cent declined admission and 65 per cent said it was due to cost. Several analysts suggest that the urban poor need some form of health-care safety net (Wu *et al.*, 1999). The Ministry of Civil Affairs has begun experiments with such a scheme (Chapter 2). Migrants do not have the same access to basic health services as registered residents. For example, migrants to Shanghai and Chengdu use reproductive health services much less than permanent residents (Zhan *et al.*, 2000; Tian *et al.*, 1999).

Changing Patterns of Entitlement to Health Services

This section discusses how economic changes are affecting entitlements to social benefits. Entitlements are legitimate claims by individuals on the state or other institutions. A government's ability to honour entitlements is an important source of its legitimacy. Attempts to renegotiate entitlements involve political costs. China has assigned entitlements to social benefits mostly on the basis of a person's place of residence and the kind of work they do (Wong, 1998; Solinger, 1999; Bloom, 2001).

One aspect of the transition to a market economy has been the transformation of entitlements from informal claims on employers and government into ownership of assets and rules-based rights to government assistance. Two examples are the sale of housing to long-term employees at subsidized prices and the establishment of safety nets for people living below a defined poverty line. These changes are institutionalizing new patterns of differential access to social benefits (Wang, 2001).

A paper by the Project on Social Development in China at the Chinese Academy of Social Sciences (CASS, 1998) argues that China has reached the 'middle stage' of its reforms. It argues that 'difficult questions of patterns of interest' must be addressed and that successful reforms will depend on the management of the 'readjustment of basic interest relationships'. It stresses the need to ensure that all social groups benefit from development and identifies the following interests to be reconciled during the establishment of a new social security system over the next 10–15 years:

- The very high financial burden of social benefits on state-owned enterprises compared to other categories of enterprise;
- The difference in social benefits between urban and rural residents and the rapid growth of employment in enterprises outside the cities;
- The differences in earnings and access to benefits between well-developed and under-developed regions and the need for substantial investment to close the gap;
- The effort by governments of rich localities to limit the outflow of tax revenue and by national government to reduce inter-regional inequality.

Li, Peilin (2002) argues that it is 'essential for future sustainable development in China to bring about a reasonable order of social stratification with the aid of the legal system'. He goes on to say that 'without a legal economy there will be no moral economy' (p.45). This is an argument for the establishment of rules-based entitlements appropriate to new (socially legitimate) patterns of social stratification. The following sections discuss the challenge of balancing the need to honour existing claims and the need to create new rules of entitlement appropriate to present and future social arrangements (Zhang, 2002).

Balancing Claims of Rural and Urban Residents

The household registration system, which limits the movement of people, underpins a sharp divide between rural and urban residents (Cook and White, 1998; Chan and Zhang, 1999). Rural residents have been entitled to little more than access to the means of agricultural production. This translates into a right to a fair share of land in a locality. The government makes modest fiscal transfers to poor areas and organizes national poverty reduction programmes. Local governments and collective bodies finance basic support for the poorest people.

In contrast, urban residents have been entitled to a wide range of benefits in what Solinger (1999) calls 'the urban public goods regime'. Urban registration is associated with much higher levels of entitlement to benefits. For example, Wang and Zuo (1999) confirmed that only a small proportion of Shanghai's migrants had health insurance.

The clear demarcation between urban and rural entitlements has begun to erode. Rural-to-urban migrants work in a variety of settings (Solinger, 1999). The urban workforce is stratified into categories of registration such as fully registered, newly registered, temporary residents and unregistered peasants (Chan and Zhang, 1999). These categories have quite different entitlements to benefits.

There are plans to overhaul the household registration system. Some cities have phased out the differentiation between urban and rural registration between localities within their boundaries. Guangdong and Jiangsu Provinces have removed the boundary between rural and urban residents, so that people can relocate anywhere within the province. Elsewhere, the definition of the urban population and hence those entitled to jobs and better social benefits continues to be highly contested. The labour market is much more complex than it was. There is no longer a simple identity between urban registration and non-agricultural employment. The challenge is to create a rules-based system of entitlements that reflects this complexity (CASS, 1998).

Changing Patterns of Entitlement Amongst Urban Residents

City dwellers were entitled to a job under the command economy (Leung, 1995). Entitlements to most benefits are still based on place of employment. The government and state-owned enterprises provide comprehensive packages of benefits. Other employers provide less generous benefits. Local governments also finance benefits for specific social groups. Their health departments fund medical care for veterans of the liberation war and certain retired government officials. Departments of civil affairs provide a basic living allowance to people whose household income falls below a locally determined minimum living standard.

Urban residents have a strong sense of entitlement to social security and services. The report by the Chinese Academy of Social Sciences highlights this: 'the elimination of workplace security in cities means the elimination of employees' rights and benefits. Widespread resistance to this measure is therefore a matter of course' (CASS, 1998, p.89). Croll (1999) and Howell (1997) cite outbreaks of civil disturbance and strikes in defence of jobs, pensions and health insurance as evidence of the strength of feeling on this issue. Government strategies for social sector reform have been strongly influenced by these attitudes.

The transition to a market economy has led to changes in the pattern of entitlements (Selden and Lou, 1997). There has been a shift from permanent employment to fixed-term contracts. Between 1986 and 1997 the proportion of employees of state enterprises on short-term contracts rose from 7 per cent to 51.6 per cent (Hussain, 1999). Enterprises now have the right to lay off workers. Urban residents are no longer guaranteed a job. Government has acted to prevent large-scale unemployment (Wong, 1999). It has encouraged people to retire; it has pressured government institutions, such as hospitals, to increase their workforce; it has subsidized loss-making enterprises; and it has established a system of unemployment benefits.

A growing number of urban residents work for neither government, nor state-owned enterprises (Table 1.3). The different categories of enterprise vary considerably in the age and sex of their employees and the levels of pay and benefits they provide. Government institutions and state-owned enterprises tend to have older employees with well-established entitlements to benefits. Their new employees are more likely to be on short-term contracts, associated with fewer benefits. Some of these new employees may not have full urban registration.

Other categories of enterprise tend to be newer and to employ younger people. Successful companies pay high salaries but provide fewer long-term benefits. The author visited a joint venture which employed mostly young female migrants from surrounding counties. The company provided excellent maternity benefits but was not building a fund for future health care needs.

Older workers and those who have been in the same job for a long time are more likely to have health insurance. A survey of 22 cities in 1992 by Hu *et al.* (1999) found that older workers are more likely to have health insurance than younger ones. A survey in Shanghai found that 47 per cent of those hired within the past ten years had health insurance, compared with 80 per cent of those hired before then (Wang and Zuo, 1999).

State-owned enterprises are finding it increasingly difficult to finance health insurance. Over a third of the workforce of some enterprises are retired. Their health benefits can be costly. Many state-owned enterprises are losing money and cannot afford their employees' medical benefits. Late payment or non-payment of medical costs is common.

The government is transferring the organization of social security benefits from employers to newly created social security institutions. One of the government's challenges in formulating strategies for social security reform is to reconcile the interests of different age cohorts and categories of enterprise and people with varying registration status. Selden and Lou (1997) put this forward as an explanation of the difficulty it is having in establishing a uniform pension scheme. They suggest that compliance rates below 100 per cent reflect the unwillingness of new enterprises to contribute to a fund from which the main beneficiaries will be current pensioners. Yu and Ren (1998) make a similar point about health insurance. They suggest that a company's decision to join a local scheme is influenced by the size of contributions, the age of their workforce and whether they own a health facility.

Reconciling Entitlements of Different Age Cohorts

The government is managing two simultaneous processes in creating new social security arrangements. It is attempting to establish a system of rules-based entitlements that people trust. It is also endeavouring to finance current entitlements. In doing so it has to balance claims by different age cohorts.

Policy debates mostly concern the broad shape of future social security arrangements. They tend to reflect the views of national ministries and heads of provincial governments (Liu and Bloom, 2002). Implementation is strongly influenced by local government, social groups with political influence, and enterprises. Young and old, men and women, and employees of different categories of enterprise have different interests. The following paragraphs discuss policy and implementation in turn. They focus on pensions, because a considerable amount of work has been done on this ,topic. However, similar issues arise with health insurance, since a high proportion of claims are by the elderly.

Discussions about pensions have focused on the arrangements to be established after a 10- to 15-year transition. China's future system has to balance social solidarity against the need to take differences in pay into account (CASS, 2000). The government advocates the establishment of a basic pension funded by government and enterprises, individual pension accounts financed by individuals and employers, and voluntary private top-up pensions.[6] The idea is to permit the size of pensions to vary with salaries whilst ensuring that the entire eligible population has a basic pension. It leaves unresolved, issues regarding who is eligible for a basic pension and how it should be financed.

The great differences in average earnings between localities are a major barrier to the creation of a unified pension system. The provision of a uniform basic pension assumes a relatively integrated labour market. Otherwise residents of poor localities would receive a higher share of local salaries and residents of rich localities would receive a lower one. These differences would be heightened if coverage were extended to employees of rural-based enterprises and rural-to-urban migrants. This would leave residents of expensive cities relatively unprotected and either put a substantial financial burden on governments of poor localities or imply substantial resource transfers between localities.

The most difficult questions regarding the basic pension concern finance. Should each locality fund basic pensions for its own residents? Or should contributions be related to a local government's ability to pay? If local governments are fully responsible, they have to reconcile the need to finance pensions for city dwellers against calls on their resources to provide benefits to farmers. Richer governments could be required to subsidise pensions in poor areas. The advantage of this form of redistribution has to be weighed against its impact on the willingness of governments to transfer funds to poor rural counties. Discussions about the financial basis for pensions are closely linked to broader discussions about the reform of public finance.

China is reforming its social security system late in the demographic transition. It has to finance current claims for pensions (and health insurance) whilst building up pension funds. It also has to address the problems of the majority of the elderly, who live outside the cities and have no pension entitlements.

The government subsidizes pensions. The Ministry of Finance transferred CNY17 billion to cover pension shortfalls in 1999 and CNY20 billion in 2000 (Ma and Zhai, 2001). This was a major transfer of resources to urban residents. One possible explanation of government's unwillingness to translate pension entitlements into clear financial commitments is that it wants to leave open the possibility of renegotiating entitlements as the situation changes. For example, it is keeping the retirement age low to reduce open unemployment, but the long-term sustainability of funded pensions depends on raising the retirement age. Urban dwellers will ultimately have to come to terms with competition from rural-based enterprises, which will provide very modest pensions to their employees. Present entitlements to pensions are fuzzy and arrangements for financing them are *ad hoc*. This gives stakeholders time to adjust their expectations to changing economic realities.

The lack of clear rules has costs. It contributes to feelings of insecurity. This encourages stakeholders to seek ways to minimize short-term financial burdens. For example, municipalities with profitable firms and/or younger populations have resisted arrangements that would involve substantial transfers of resources to other localities (Wong, 1999). New enterprises have attempted to avoid excessive liabilities for pensions and health insurance by keeping out of new schemes. Some enterprises may have been set up outside municipal boundaries for this reason.

Some *ad hoc* measures have had a deleterious effect on the establishment of a rules-based system. In theory, the creation of individual accounts provides a means to build up a funded pension scheme. In practice, schemes have used funds from individual accounts to finance existing pensions. Ma and Zhai (2001) estimate that schemes withdrew CNY1 billion from individual accounts for this purpose in 2000. Little is known about how young workers view this use of their pension contributions. These examples illustrate the difficulties associated with managing simultaneously the establishment of a new social security system and the funding of existing claims to benefits. One requires transparency and the other requires opaqueness.

It may be helpful to separate the issues of financing existing entitlements and establishing actuarially sound social security institutions. There are several options for financing existing pensions (CASS, 2000; Wang, X., 2001; Ma and Zhai, 2001). Young workers and their employers could be asked to make higher contributions to social security schemes than would be required to build up their own entitlements, or they could be required to pay higher taxes. Local governments could issue bonds with promises to repay out of future taxes. Assets could be transferred to the social security fund in the form of ownership of a company, shares in a company or cash earned by selling a company. The latter options represent a translation of fuzzy pension entitlements into ownership of funded assets. They would institutionalize differences in entitlement between social groups. Government has to reconcile the interests of pensioners and of social groups that do not have work-related benefits in establishing levels of pensions to be funded this way.

Health insurance is more complex than pensions. The cost of pensions is directly related to the number of people above retirement age and the rules defining the size of payment. The cost of health benefits depends on the many factors that determine needs and expectations of services to address them. However, the same issues apply with regard to the need simultaneously to finance existing claims and establish rules-based insurance schemes.

The Policy Process in China

China's strategy for transition management has strongly influenced the policy process. The government system is highly decentralized (World Bank, 2002). Each level of government collects taxes and transfers some to higher levels, according to complex and changing rules. Local governments have a great deal of autonomy in deciding how to use their revenue. City governments have substantial sources of revenue in addition to taxes. Many local administrations own enterprises that pay profits or management fees. They also own land and collect ground rent. Local governments can use this 'extra-budgetary revenue' as they wish.

This decentralization has had two important consequences. It has led to growing differences in the resources available to local governments: some have very substantial revenues and others can barely pay salaries. It has also given local governments a lot of control over their own resources, and has limited the capacity of higher levels of government to do so.

The government is organized in a number of vertical structures that extend from national to local administrative levels (Bloom and Fang, 2003). Each level of government more or less replicates the structure at national level. Many commissions and ministries have health-related mandates for planning, service provision, finance, regulation and accountability (Table 1.5).

Table 1.5 Government organizations with an influence on health

Ministry of commission	Principal health-related functions
Planning	
State Development Planning Commission	Responsible for five-year plan and also special public sector investment programmes.
Ministry of Finance	Annual budget.
Service provision	
Ministry of Health	Responsible for the performance of health institutions.
State Family Planning Commission	Implementation of family planning policy.
Ministry of National Defence, Ministry of Railways and other sector ministries	Health facilities that serve sector employees or are owned by work units under the sector.
Finance	
Ministry of Health	Partial subsidies of public health facilities. Health insurance for government employees.
Ministry of Labour and Social Security	Urban health insurance.
Ministry of Civil Affairs	Safety net for the poor.
Regulation and accountability	
Ministry of Health	Enforcement of health-related regulations.
Ministry of Personnel	Management of civil servants and cadres. Oversight of public sector employment of skilled workers.
Ministry of Labour and Social Security	Oversight of public sector employment of semi-skilled and unskilled workers.
Price Bureau of State Development Planning Commission	Setting prices of services and health-related commodities.
State Drug Management and Monitoring Bureau	Enforcement of regulation of pharmaceutical sector. Oversight of government pharmaceutical companies and distribution systems.
Auditing Administration	Financial audit.

The State Development Planning Commission oversees the formulation and implementation of five-year regional health plans and the Ministry of Finance is responsible for annual budgets and monitoring of financial management.

The Ministry of Health is responsible for government health facilities. Several other ministries 'own' health facilities or oversee enterprises that do so and the State Family Planning Commission has a network of service delivery institutions. The Ministry of Health provides annual grants to government health institutes and facilities and it pays contributions to local health insurance schemes for government employees. The Ministry of Labour and Social Security is responsible for urban health insurance and the Ministry of Civil Affairs funds safety nets for the poor.

The Ministry of Health oversees the performance of its facilities and regulates private providers. The State Drug Management and Monitoring Bureau is responsible for ensuring that drugs are effective and safe. The Ministry of Personnel manages civil servants and also skilled workers in public employment. The Ministry of Labour and Social Security plays a similar role regarding semi-skilled and unskilled workers. The Price Bureau, under the State Development Planning Commission, sets prices for health services and health-related commodities. The Ministry of Civil Affairs oversees the elected village committees and social organizations. The Auditing Administration establishes rules for financial audit.

The organization of the government into parallel vertical channels has advantages and disadvantages. It has established very effective preventive programmes that have continued to operate despite the many changes that have taken place. The separation of the demand and supply sides between the Ministry of Labour and Social Security and the Ministry of Health may reduce the tendency of government health facilities to give more weight to the needs of health workers than of the people they serve. However, it has created difficulties in coordination between agencies and even between departments within a single ministry. No single institution has overall responsibility for coordinating health-related activities. This has made it difficult to formulate coherent development strategies.

China's leaders describe the management of reform as crossing a stream whilst feeling for the stones. This is a graphic metaphor for the tentative nature of decision-making in China (Lieberthal and Oksenberg, 1988). The usual process involves the gradual construction of consensus at national and provincial levels in favour of a new policy (Liu and Bloom, 2002). The initial government proclamations often state general principles, rather than specific and enforceable regulations. These general statements may evolve into specific rules, or they may be altered or disregarded.

The evolution of a policy statement into a change in the rules of behaviour for local governments and economic actors is lengthy and complex. Local governments translate national policies into local regulations. Some localities may ignore a policy or implement it unenthusiastically. While the evolution is taking place there is a great deal of ambiguity about what constitutes acceptable behaviour. The approach to transition management has enabled actors to adapt to rapidly changing circumstances without excessive disruption. It has also made it possible for different localities to evolve different institutional arrangements.

One strategy favoured by policy-makers is to ask a small number of local governments to pilot test an institutional innovation. If the test goes well, other localities are encouraged to emulate it. Eventually, the innovative approach may be institutionalized into national guidelines and into law. The government has pursued this approach with regard to the reform of health insurance. One of the study cities, Nantong, is amongst the 57 cities that have been testing a new kind of city-wide health insurance since the late 1990s. That is why the Ministry of Health suggested that we include it in this study.

Notes

1   *China Statistical Yearbook*, 2001, Tables 3.1 and 3.4.
2   *China Statistical Yearbook*, 2001, Tables 10.3 and 10.9.
3   *China Statistical Yearbook*, 2001, Table 3.9.
4   *China Statistical Yearbook*, 2001, Table 10.5.
5   *China Statistical Yearbook*, 2001, Table 5.1.
6   State Council Documents No. 26, 1997 and No. 42, 2000.

Chapter 2

Introduction to the Urban Health System and Review of Reform Initiatives

Shenglan Tang and Qingyue Meng

This chapter first provides a brief introduction to the evolution of urban health services and health insurance schemes which have been developed since the foundation of the People's Republic. It then describes and discusses the reforms of urban health services and health insurance schemes which have been initiated during the two decades since the economic reform launched in the late 1970s and their implications for equity and efficiency in urban China.

Evolution of Urban Health Services

The evolution of urban health services in China over the past half-century can be divided into three periods: from the founding of the People's Republic in 1949 to the eve of the Great Cultural Revolution in 1965; the years in which the Great Cultural Revolution was taking place (1966–77); and from the beginning of the economic reform in 1978 to the present.

The Period Between 1949 and 1965

Mainland China inherited a poorly developed health sector in 1949 when the People's Republic was established by the Chinese Communist Party (Horn, 1969). The major providers of medical care were the practitioners of traditional Chinese medicine who used a combination of herbal medicine, acupuncture and other traditional methods to treat patients. The relatively small number of doctors of Western medicine worked mainly in the urban hospitals.

In 1951 and 1952 the First and Second National Health Conferences sponsored by the State Council of the new government were held and the following health policies were announced (Fu, 1953):

- Medicine must serve the working people (workers, peasants and soldiers);
- Preventive programmes must be given priority over curative care;
- Health services must integrate the services of practitioners of traditional Chinese medicine and Western medicine;
- Health work must be integrated with mass movements.

From the early 1950s to 1965, before the beginning of the Great Cultural Revolution, existing facilities were renovated and new 'people's hospitals' and other preventive health facilities were built in each city and urban district. The network of urban health services was expanded. The number of hospitals run by the urban health sector of China rose from 275 in 1950 to 1,421 in 1965 (Ministry of Health, 1989). In the cities a large number of 'street' or community hospitals and clinics (mainly for out-patient services) were built. Paramedics were trained to serve at community clinics, acting as the first line of health services. Some industrial sectors, such as mining, railways and telecommunications, and military organizations established around 1,500 hospitals by 1965. Most of these hospitals were located in the urban areas, serving the employees and dependants of these industries. In addition, almost every government institution, enterprise and school had a health clinic which provided very basic curative and preventive services.

Training capacity expanded rapidly over the period. The number of graduates of medical and pharmaceutical schools grew from 1,314 in 1949 to 22,027 in 1965. As a result, the number of doctors of Western medicine in China increased five-fold and the number of pharmacists rose from virtually zero to 8,000 in 1965. Most of the doctors and pharmacists were employed by the urban hospitals and other health facilities, although efforts were made by the government to deploy more health professionals in the countryside.

From the early 1950s the government organized a number of mass campaigns to tackle the problem of communicable, and often preventable, diseases. These campaigns were led by the State Patriotic Health Campaign Committee and its branches at every level of government. The Communist Party of China played an important role in mobilizing people to carry out public health and sanitation-related activities. Campaigns were also organized against specific diseases. For example, thousands of people were trained to recognize the symptoms and signs of sexually transmitted diseases, encourage treatment and administer antibiotics. Another mass campaign aimed to control schistosomiasis, a parasitic illness acquired from working barefoot in contaminated water. During the early 1960s, the Ministry of Health began a programme of immunization against several common diseases.

Over the period, the responsibility for infectious disease control shifted from the Patriotic Health Campaign Committee to newly established anti-epidemic stations (AESs) at district/county, regional and provincial levels. In 1950, only 61 AESs existed in China. By 1995, about 2,500 AESs had been set up at county/district and city levels. They had three main functions: communicable disease prevention and control, including surveillance and control of endemic and epidemic infectious diseases, and immunizations; environmental hygiene and food safety; and health education and promotion.

In addition to AESs, a number of maternal and child health (MCH) centres were established in both rural counties and urban districts/cities from 1950 to 1965. The number of MCH centres increased from around 350 in 1950 to 2,700 in 1965. The main purpose of setting up MCH centres in these counties, districts and cities was to strengthen maternal and child care services and thus reduce high infant and maternal mortality rates.

The development of the health sector, particularly in urban China, mainly followed the model adopted by the former Soviet Union during the 1950s and early 1960s before the end of friendship between China and the Soviet Union. Many achievements in the improvement of the health of the vast majority of the Chinese population were made during that period. However, most of the rural population in China still did not have adequate access to basic health services. Private practitioners based in small clinics at the township and county levels were the main service providers in the rural areas. At the same time, the majority of urban residents, who were covered by a government insurance scheme (GIS) and a labour insurance scheme (LIS), had the right to virtually free health care. The government still needed to address the inequalities in access to health care between the rural and urban areas.

The Period of the Great Cultural Revolution

In 1965 Chairman Mao made a famous speech criticizing the health sector for favouring the urban areas and calling for a radical change in priorities. At almost the same time Mao and his political allies within the Communist Party Committee of China launched the Great Cultural Revolution, which brought political and economic turbulence to China over the following decade.

The new Ministry of Health dominated by leftist revolutionaries began to make rural health development its priority policy. This resulted in the training of large numbers of 'barefoot doctors' – part-farmers/part-doctors – to play a key role in the provision of rural health care, the construction of rural health facilities, and the establishment of rural cooperative medical schemes to provide funds for rural health services.

An important health sector goal during the Great Cultural Revolution was reduction of the inequality in the numbers of health workers between urban and rural areas. Many training and research centres in the urban areas closed. The organization of medical training programmes such as high-level medical education was restructured. A five-year medical training programme for medical and public health doctors was reduced to three years. Many urban hospitals sent some of their doctors to the countryside to provide the rural residents with better health care and to supervise poorly trained health workers at the rural grassroots. For example, in 1969 Gansu Province in western China decided to send 50 per cent of the doctors working in its cities to rural health facilities (Gansu Provincial Department of Health, 2000). At the same time, new medical and public health graduates were automatically assigned to rural facilities. Table 2.1 shows the consequences of the radical changes in policy for health human resources adopted over the period. The number of qualified doctors in rural areas was almost doubled within ten years, while the number of doctors in urban areas rose by only 36 per cent. The number of nurses in rural areas increased by 137 per cent, while the number in urban areas increased by only 37 per cent. Only the increase in the number of assistant doctors was greater in the urban areas than in the rural areas over the period.

Table 2.1 Increase in the number of health professionals in China, 1965–75

	Doctors		Assistant doctors		Nurses	
	Urban	Rural	Urban	Rural	Urban	Rural
1965	131,091	57,570	97,969	154,744	175,644	58,902
1975	177,790	115,192	144,849	211,250	239,972	139,573
% increase	36	100	48	37	37	137

More health facility construction took place in the rural areas while the development of urban health sector slowed down. The total number of commune (township) health centres rose from 35,733 in 1966 to 54,541 ten years later, although the number of hospitals and other health facilities at the county and upper level changed little in the same time. For example, the number of district/city hospitals managed by the health sector rose only from 1,421 in 1965 to 1,628 in 1975 (Ministry of Health, 1989). No more AESs were built in the urban areas over the period, while the number of MCH centres actually declined slightly, although no precise figure is available. However, many villages in the countryside built their own health stations staffed by barefoot doctors. By 1975 over 85 per cent of villages in the rural areas had a health station. This provided the infrastructure of the three-tier rural health care: village, commune/township and county.

While the infrastructure of the three-tier network of health care and the capacity of service provision in the rural areas were strengthened during the Great Cultural Revolution, the urban health sector, from tertiary hospitals to community health centres and clinics suffered to varying degrees. As one Chinese professor said,[1] a good referral system involving community health centres and clinics, district hospitals and tertiary/teaching hospitals in urban areas of China, which was well established in the 17 years since the founding of the People's Republic, collapsed during that period. Many qualified doctors and other health professionals left the urban areas for the countryside. As a consequence, the capacity of service provision was jeopardized and the overall quality of health care in many cities deteriorated.

In summary, the outcomes of the health sector emanating from the Great Cultural Revolution were mixed. On one hand, many health institutions and medical/pharmaceutical schools were unable to function effectively, with deleterious effects on education and research. On the other hand, the health status of the rural population in China improved dramatically, resulting from, among others, the deployment of qualified doctors, the training of barefoot doctors and the development of rural cooperative medical schemes.

Organization and Financing of the Urban Health Sector

The basic structure of the present urban health services was fully established by the 1970s. This section first introduces how the health sector and relevant government agencies have been organized and are functioning, followed by a discussion of financing of the urban health sector in general.

The Ministry of Health, under the authority of the State Council, provides overall leadership to the health sector. Each level of district/county and higher local government has a health department which is answerable to the government at the same level and to the health department of the next higher level (Figure 2.1). Often, the prefecture level[2] is not a separate level of government, but simply functions as a regional department of the provincial government.

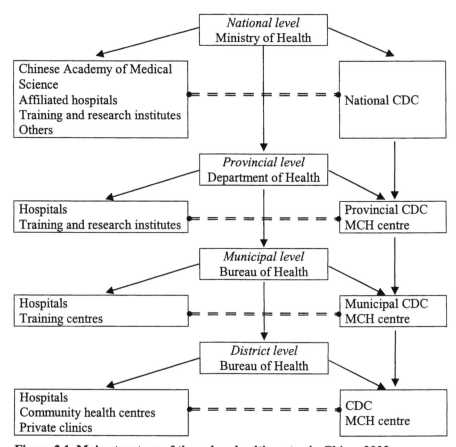

Figure 2.1 Main structure of the urban health sector in China, 2003

At each level there are hospitals, preventive services (e.g. AESs and MCH centres), and medical and health training institutions (e.g. medical colleges and health schools), a majority of which are directly supervised by the corresponding health department. In recent years, more and more training institutions have been handed over from the health department to the education department at the same level of local government, as part of a restructuring of the public sector in China. Meanwhile, as part of its reform of the organization of the health sector, central government has been trying to gather all the preventive service institutions under one big umbrella – the Centre for Disease Control and Prevention (CDC). As a result, the CDC, which was built on the previous Chinese Academy of Preventive Medicine, has been set up at the national level. All provinces and cities have been required to establish their own CDCs by merging the previous AESs and other infectious disease control centres and institutions. Within the national CDC there is a national MCH centre, but almost all MCH centres at provincial level and below are still independent from their parallel CDCs.

In some urban areas there are many hospitals and clinics which are owned and run by different industrial sectors, large state-owned enterprises (SOEs), or military organizations. In 1995 these hospitals and health facilities had about half a million hospital beds, while the health sector managed by the Ministry of Health and departments of health at different administrative levels had about 1 million hospital beds. These hospitals hired 1.1 million health professionals, while the health sector had around 2.5 million (Ministry of Health, 1996). Although these hospitals provide their services mainly to their employees and their family members, they also open to the public generally.

In addition, the General Office of the National Patriotic Health Campaign Commission, which is part of the Ministry of Health, is responsible for leading the patriotic health campaigns. The National Patriotic Health Campaign Commission has branches at each level of local government which are usually located within the health department.

Parallel to the Ministry of Health at national level and the health departments of local governments, there is another government agency called the National Family Planning Commission whose mandate is mainly to develop population policies aimed at controlling the rapid rise of the Chinese population over the past century, particularly in rural areas. The political status of the Commission is slightly higher than that of the Ministry of Health, since population control in China has been placed higher on the political agenda by central government. At each level of local government there is a family planning committee often headed by the governor of the local governments. In addition, many rural townships and counties have established family planning stations which are providing services related to contraception and other reproductive health matters. Most urban districts have also set up stations of this kind to provide contraceptive and counselling services to the public including rural-to-urban migrants. The family planning stations in many urban districts and rural counties often compete with the MCH centres in the provision of maternal and other reproductive care services.

The Ministry of Labour and Social Security was set up in 1997. One of its mandates is to develop the social security system including urban health insurance schemes in China. More detailed information about the Ministry and urban health insurance schemes are provided later in this chapter.

The Ministry of Civil Affairs and the civil affairs departments at provincial and lower levels provide another vertical system whose aim is to protect the poor and vulnerable groups and set up social safety nets for the Chinese population. Although the system provides financial and other support to the poor in both urban and rural areas, it does not have a sizeable budget earmarked to help those in the need seeking health care. Having successfully established an income support scheme in all Chinese cities over the past decade, the Ministry of Civil Affairs and particularly the departments of civil affairs in some rich cities, for example in Shanghai and Guangdong, have started to support the urban poor and vulnerable groups in health care, through medical financial assistance schemes for the poor. However, the support given to the needy has so far been very limited.

The supply and use of both Western and Chinese medicine and drugs is one of the key elements of health care in China. The State Drug Administrative Bureau was set up to develop drug-related regulations, approve the use of new drugs and monitor the use of all drugs in China. Initially the Bureau was established within the Ministry of Health but has now become an independent government agency. At the provincial and lower levels, respective bureaux responsible for drug administration were also set up to carry out the same functions.

The financing of the urban health sector has been complex in China and it is not easy to put together a complete picture. There have been three major financing mechanisms in the urban health sector of China: government health budgets, insurance schemes arising from waged/salary employment and direct user payments. Their relative importance has changed over time, which we will discuss later in this chapter. There are considerable regional differences in per capita health expenditures in China, due largely to significant differences in economic development between the regions

The financing of urban public hospitals has been evolving since the founding of the People's Republic in 1949.[3] In the 1950s all the revenues generated in public hospitals (mainly through direct user payment) were handed over to the treasury departments of local government and the recurrent expenditures of the hospitals were fully covered by government health grants. The process of hospital accounting was very complicated and difficult to manage. From 1960 to the late 1970s, 'gap budgeting' was introduced to health facilities, especially hospitals, which should be capable of generating considerable revenues. The principle of this system was that health budgetary allocations to such institutions should be used only to fill in the gap between their essential expenditures and the finance they raised. There were variants of the system, with different elements of the budget allocations being made on a fixed basis. In general, the financial support from the government should cover at least the costs of salaries of the hospital staff. For example, the total income from government health budgets in 1979 accounted for 135 per cent of the salary/wage costs of hospital staff in public hospitals. In addition, the government also took major responsibility for capital development, such as constructing new buildings and purchasing large or high-tech medical equipment. From the early 1950s to the late 1970s, the price of medical care services provided by public hospitals was set at a level far below the level of recurrent costs. In other words, user fees directly paid out of the pockets of people not covered by any health insurance were not very high.

There was another financial mechanism called full-range budgeting, which was applied mainly to preventive health institutes, for example, AESs, and MCH centres, from the 1950s to the 1970s. These institutes were providing mainly preventive services that were unlikely to generate much income. Under this system the institutes received grants from the finance departments of local governments, mostly at the same level, which could cover the costs of salary/wages and operations. Any revenues earned would revert to the government.

In summary, the structure of the urban health sector, consisting of hospitals, preventive health institutions and training centres, had been well established by the end of the 1970s, although some of the functions and performance of these institutions were negatively affected by the Great Cultural Revolution from the mid-1960s to the late 1970s. The financing of the urban health sector, particularly public hospitals, experienced several changes over the period.

Urban Health Insurance Schemes

After the founding of the People's Republic in 1949, the Chinese government set up two work-related health insurance schemes in the urban areas: the Government Insurance Scheme (GIS) and the Labour Insurance Scheme (LIS). The GIS originated in the old liberated zone controlled by the Communist Party of China in the mid-1930s. It was officially established after the State Council issued a document entitled 'Implementation Method of GIS for State Employees' in August 1952. Its beneficiaries included civil servants, university students and retired veterans. The dependants of these beneficiaries were never covered by GIS, although some places allowed individual institutions to use the budget for employee welfare/benefits to subsidize the costs of medical care for direct dependants. The financing source for the GIS were the finance departments of central or local governments, as part of annual government budget. A fixed amount of money per person was allocated by the finance department to the GIS management office, which was often physically located in the local government health bureau that managed the fund. From the late 1970s the allocated GIS funds could not fully cover employees' medical costs (Gu and Tang, 1995) and it was not uncommon for institutions to use their own revenues to supplement the costs of medical care for their employees.

The LIS was formally established in 1951 when the State Council of the Chinese government issued 'The Regulations for Labour Insurance of People's Republic of China'. Its beneficiaries were the employees working in SOEs and their direct dependants. The LIS provided full coverage of medical costs for employees and partial coverage for their dependants. The government required collectively owned enterprises (COEs) to implement the same policies for the LIS as the SOEs. The LIS also covered medical care and other services, such as maternity leave benefits. The funding for the LIS came from the benefit/welfare budget of each enterprise. On average, expenditure on the LIS accounted for 11–14 per cent of the gross wage/salary costs of the enterprises before the early 1990s.

Until the early 1990s, the GIS and the LIS covered, fully or partially, about half of China's urban population. A recent national health service survey showed that the coverage of health insurance declined significantly from 54 per cent of the urban population in 1993 to 39 per cent in 1998 (Gao and Tang, 2000). Table 2.2 shows the percentage change of health insurance coverage among the urban Chinese population between 1993 and 1998. There has been a large increase in the proportion of the population who are not covered by any health insurance and have to pay out of pocket for health services under circumstances in which the cost of medical care has risen rapidly.

Table 2.2 Percentage change in health insurance coverage of urban Chinese population, 1993–8

	GIS/LIS (%)	Commercial insurance (%)	Others* (%)	No insurance (%)
1993	53.5	0.3	19.0	27.3
1998	38.9	3.3	17.4	44.1

*Others include a variety of health plans enjoyed by those living in the urban areas (including rural cooperative medical schemes for rural migrants and financial subsidies for dependants of LIS beneficiaries).

The decrease in urban health insurance coverage can be attributed to the interplay of four factors. The first factor is the continuous urbanization over the past two decades. In 1978 only 20 per cent of the Chinese population were regarded as urban; by the year 2000 about 36.1 per cent were living in urban areas (National Bureau of Statistics, 2001). Many rural counties, where the percentage of the population covered by the GIS and LIS was low, have been upgraded to urban cities. Second, more adults in the urban areas were unemployed in 1998 than in 1993.[4] A vast majority of these people lost work-related benefits, including health insurance, when they lost jobs or were laid off. Third, many enterprises and local governments have experienced financial difficulties in paying for medical care for their employees, undermining the financial viability of both the GIS and the LIS. Lastly, a significant number of rural emigrants are now living and working in the economically developed urban areas, although there are no official figures reported.

The financing and management problems of the GIS and LIS are nothing less than alarming. While the number of beneficiaries covered by the two schemes rose from 92 million in 1978 to 153 million in 1997, the total amount of GIS and LIS expenditure increased from CNY3.16 billion to CNY77.37 billion over the same period (Cai, 2001). Even accounting for inflation, the escalation of medical care costs for the GIS and LIS over the 20-year period is still striking. Medical care accounted for 9.1 per cent of wage/salary costs in 1997, much higher than the figure of 5.8 per cent in 1978. Not surprisingly, both governments and enterprises suffered formidable difficulties in paying these medical bills.

It became apparent that the government and many enterprises could no longer afford to fund the GIS and LIS as they once did. A major problem was the lack of an appropriate mechanism for financing the GIS and LIS. Although the central government provided guidelines on the allocation of financial resource for the GIS and LIS to the local governments and enterprises, the implementation of these guidelines was often ineffective. This was largely owing to a decentralized fiscal system, in addition to the financial difficulties faced by many institutions. GIS expenditure in 1996, for example, clearly demonstrated the degree of seriousness of these financing constraints. Total GIS expenditure in that year was CNY16.43 billion. However, the fund allocated by central and local governments for the scheme was only about CNY11.02 billion, accounting for only 67 per cent of total expenditure. Because of directives from the central government, public hospitals in China used their revenues (CNY3.18 billion) to pay for part of the GIS expenditure on behalf of central or local governments, accounting for 19.1 per cent of total GIS expenditure in 1996. Meanwhile, GIS management offices still owed CNY753 million (4.6 per cent of total GIS expenditure) to their designated hospitals. The financial shortfall was covered by public institutions within the GIS and their employees (via co-payment arrangements).

What happened? First, the regulations of GIS and LIS required governments (central and local) and enterprises to pay almost the entire medical care costs incurred by their employees. They acted as 'third party payer', but did not have any capacity for monitoring and supervising the provision of services. Nor did they have any mechanisms and means to influence the behaviour of service providers. Providers benefited significantly from the fee-for-service payment method used because there was no mechanism for evaluating whether the services and procedures offered were appropriate or necessary, let alone cost-effective. For example, the price structure of pharmaceuticals allowed for mark-ups of 15 per cent at both wholesale and retail levels. Profits were therefore generated from drug prescription and the use of more expensive drugs. As a result, 52 per cent of health spending in the early 1990s was for prescription drugs. And while there was waste resulting from excessive and superfluous services, many of the urban population, particularly those working in loss-making enterprises or not covered by any health insurance, were not able to access even the most basic health care. It was a situation of feast and famine.

Another problem was that both the GIS and the LIS had limited capacity for risk-sharing, let alone combined purchasing power. Each institution or enterprise was responsible for its own beneficiaries. There was no financial pooling and risk-sharing between the institutions within the GIS or between the enterprises within the LIS. Therefore, a catastrophic illness among a few employees could bankrupt the health plan of a smaller enterprise. And by functioning as independent entities, enterprises lost valuable cost-saving opportunities such as collective bargaining, economy of scale and purchasing power. So while institutions and enterprises with sound fiscal status could provide their beneficiaries with very good medical care packages, those with poor fiscal status, or with a substantial number of retirees to take care of, may have provided only very limited coverage.

It had become apparent to both the central and local governments that the GIS and LIS needed to be reformed. Since then, local and central governments, acting either in concert or separately, have tried various experimental reforms. These have all aimed at transforming the two crippled insurance schemes into more equitable, affordable and sustainable ventures.

Reforms of Urban Health Services and Health Insurance

This section briefly introduces the reform of urban health services in general and hospitals in particular. It then discusses reforms of the GIS and LIS since the economic reform.

Reforming Urban Health Services

China launched its economic reform in 1978, immediately after the ending of the Great Cultural Revolution. The overall objective of the economic reform was to speed up the development of China's economy by decentralizing decision-making from central government to local government and individual institutions, and by liberating labour and product markets. All these changes have inevitably made the health sector adapt to the changing environment in which public hospitals and other health facilities are operating. This section looks at the areas of reform related to the financing of public hospitals and other health facilities, the decentralization of health services management, price setting for health services, and regional health planning; and to the impact of these reforms on service providers. The following section discusses the reform of urban health insurance schemes and its impacts, mainly on service users.

One of the main components of economic reform in China is fiscal decentralization, which was introduced at the beginning of the 1980s. Under the fiscal decentralization the authority to decide on sectoral allocation was delegated to provincial and lower level governments, although the higher levels of the health service remained in a technical supervisory relationship with the levels below. In other words, local governments could decide how much money to allocate to support health care in their localities, that is, how big a grant to allocate to their local hospitals and other health facilities. For most local governments in China, the development of health care has not been a priority over the past two decades. Developing the local economy has always been given a higher priority than health care and other social services. As a result, the proportion of income from government has declined significantly and become less important to hospital finance since the economic reform. It accounted for only 8.7 per cent on average of hospital revenues in 2000 (Table 2.3). A financial responsibility system was introduced in many places, which required hospitals and other health facilities to generate as much revenue as possible by charging fees for their services. This has pushed the hospitals into increasing their charges to patients to cover operational costs, which have been rising rapidly over the past two decades. Table 2.3 provides a clear picture of how sources of hospital income have changed over the past two decades.

Similarly, all the preventive service institutions have no longer enjoyed full-range budgeting. Most local governments have tried to cover only the cost of staff salaries, but in reality few can provide grants that can cover the staff salaries of these preventive service institutions. In 2000 central government investment in the public health system was only US$360 million out of a total budget of US$190 billion (WHO, 2003). As a consequence, managers of some of these institutions decided to provide some clinical services that could help generate revenues and make profits. Others tried to introduce charges for some preventive care or supervisory services. For example, many AESs wanted to open clinics providing STD diagnosis and treatment. Many MCH centres tried to provide more gynaecological care to their clients. As a whole, the financial responsibility system has provided health institutions with incentives to concentrate on revenue-earning activities.

Table 2.3 The composition of hospital incomes in China, 1980–2000

Items	1980	1985	1990	1995	2000
Total income (CNY100 million)	292.6	428.6	702.2	1,003.4	2,296.5
% of medical service	18.9	22.2	28.6	34.7	40.2
% of drugs	37.7	39.1	43.1	49.8	47.1
% of government subsidies	21.4	20.2	11.6	7.5	8.7
% of other source	22.1	18.6	16.7	7.9	4.0

Source: Ministry of Health (2001).

Under the fiscal decentralization and the financial responsibility system introduced to the health sector in general and to hospitals and other health facilities in particular, managers of these institutions have been given more autonomy in the management of their institutional financial and personnel affairs as well as in the provision of health services. If the health facilities have a financial surplus from their revenue-generation activities, the managers have the power to decide what proportion of the surplus can be used to pay bonuses and how much should be spent on investment for further development. With the support of their staff, they can set up a system that defines how bonuses should be paid to different levels or types of employee.

Furthermore, the health managers have a bigger say in the recruitment of new staff. They usually accept new employees only if they can contribute to the quality of services, although they sometimes have to make some political employments, such as veterans retired from military organizations. Increasingly, health professionals have been given job contracts instead of being offered permanent jobs as was the case previously. According to the new policies, the hospital management is in theory allowed to fire and hire staff. In practice, health managers may have difficulties in firing staff who perform poorly for many reasons, as reported by several studies (Liu, 2003). As a whole, human resource management in many health facilities has been improved greatly over the past two decades. For example, extra posts required in health facilities are usually based on the needs of service provision. The selection of new staff relies on defined procedures in which competition mechanisms have been applied. But many things remain to be done in order to improve the efficient use of health personnel.

In order to generate more revenue for their own health facilities, health managers have often strategically developed new services (e.g. through purchasing new high-tech equipment) which could help make profits for them. To some extent, the provision of care in many health facilities in China has been driven by profit, rather than the health service needs of the local population. One typical example is that the price of a CT scan examination was once set at a much higher level than its cost. The majority of district and higher-level hospitals in China have purchased CT scanners to make profits.

In addition, to enhance the performance of hospital departments and individual health workers, the managers of most hospitals have introduced a responsibility system. This sets out rules and methods for service and revenue targets for departments, units and individual staff and offers incentives for achieving these targets. The system developed in most hospitals was initially driven by a desire to increase revenue by encouraging doctors and other health professionals to provide more services and sell more drugs to their patients. This means that the more revenue doctors generated from the provision of services or the sale of drugs, the more bonus they could get in their monthly pay. Such an incentive did increase labour productivity. However, it has great implications for the cost and quality of health care. Over-prescription and overuse of high-tech diagnosis and treatment have been commonly observed in many hospitals and even in preventive service institutions. In recent years, these problems have been recognized by the government and some hospital managers. Hence, some measures to improve the quality of services, including patient satisfaction, have been brought into the responsibility system in many hospitals which used to focus only on revenues and staff workloads.

Price reform
One aim of the economic reform launched in the late 1970s was to establish a so-called socialist market economy in which prices reflected the cost of production. Prices which had been frozen since the mid-1960s were raised and private markets were permitted to flourish (Fan, 1989). However, the political leadership in China wished to avoid too rapid a rise in the price of consumer goods, which could provoke resistance, especially in the urban areas. The changing pattern of prices (i.e. a proportion of total retail sales being at market prices) over the past two decades has reflected this compromise.

As said above, before economic reform the prices of health services and drugs were set at a very low level by the government so that the vast majority of the population could afford them. The Chinese government started to reform the prices of health services from the early 1980s. The main purpose of the price reform was to let new prices reflect non-labour production costs and make service providers financially viable with limited financial support from the government grants. Under these circumstances, a new health care pricing system was established to provide guidelines for setting and regulating prices for health care and pharmaceutical products and other relevant products, and for methods used to set and adjust prices. The State Development Planning Commission is responsible for defining principles for setting health service prices, in collaboration with the Ministries of Health and Finance. Provincial or municipal government agencies, led by the Department of Price Administration, establish local fee schedules according to the local situation. Usually, official fee schedules for defined service items are published periodically (prices of drugs are not included in the fee schedule). There has been a great variation across different provinces and regions in the number of fee items, ranging from 2,500 to 6,000 in 2000. The method of setting prices is cost-based after taking out the government subsidies for basic health care, implying that fee rates and government subsides are supposed to cover all operating costs of producing a particular service or product.

The official fee schedules are compulsorily implemented according to national and provincial regulations. All public health providers must follow the fee schedules issued by their provincial or prefecture governments. Provincial and prefecture Departments of Price Administration and Health organize regulatory activities examining and monitoring hospital compliance with the official fee schedule. Hospitals that have not observed the fee schedule and overcharged patients could be punished with fines. In addition, public hospitals at and above county level are requested to set up a self-regulating pricing mechanism. A part- or full-time member of staff in each hospital should be employed to monitor the implementation of official schedules in clinical departments within the hospital. In recent years, central and local governments have also required hospitals to post the official list of major service fees in a public place in each hospital for patients' information or to use a computerized system for users to check the fee rates.

The reorganization of urban health services, called the 'development of regional health planning', is another health sector reform. Initially launched in several medium-sized cities in China in the late 1980s, many places did not take it seriously until 1996 when the central government issued an official document entitled 'Decision on Reform and Development of the Health Care System'. Three years later, the central government issued a guideline for developing regional health planning and tried to push this initiative. The driving force behind the reform was that while there was an oversupply of health resources in some urban areas, utilization of health services in urban China had gradually declined owing to a rapid rise in medical care costs and reduced insurance coverage. This is quite common in many cities where there are too many hospitals, clinics and other health facilities competing to attract patients, using different strategies and means. Most of these health facilities are run under the auspices of the health department at different levels of local governments. Some are run by medical universities and schools and others are owned and managed by different industrial sectors or large SOEs. The central government and many local governments have realized that there is an urgent need to restructure the urban health sector.

By the end of 2000, a number of provinces in China developed health resource allocation criteria for adjusting health resources. Shandong, Guangdong and Liaoning were pioneer provinces in developing and implementing new models for health resource allocation. Some municipal cities implemented regional health planning by reorganizing and redistributing health resources. As a result of this, some hospitals and clinics that provided poor quality services and thus were usually underused have been closed or merged with other hospitals. A good example is Qingdao, where several health facilities were merged and health workers were redeployed to reduce the overlap of health facilities and increase the efficiency of service provision. In addition, there has been a trend over the past decade for health facilities that were owned and run by industrial sectors or large

SOEs to be taken over by the health department of local governments as part of regional health planning reform.

All these attempts are aimed at improving the efficient use of limited health resources in different regions. In China as a whole, however, the reform initiative on regional health planning has not fully achieved its original objectives. The major reason is that in many cities it is extremely difficult to restructure health facilities that involve many sectors using different administrative mechanisms for resource allocation and management.

Reforming Urban Health Insurance

The reform of the GIS and LIS in urban China, which began in the early 1980s, consists of three distinct phases:

- Phase One: from the early 1980s to 1987;
- Phase Two: from 1988 to 1997;
- Phase Three: from 1998 to the present.

During Phase One, the reforms of the GIS and LIS can best be described as local initiatives. Several local municipal governments and enterprises developed various initiatives, trying to tackle the problem of the rapid increase in medical care costs and to increase the risk-pooling capacity and scope of the GIS and LIS. These initiatives included the following features:

- The introduction of cost-sharing mechanisms. People covered by the two health insurance schemes were required to make an out-of-pocket co-insurance payment (10–20 per cent of medical care expenditure). This was mainly aimed at controlling demand for health care and minimizing unnecessary services (by consumers least qualified to make such determinations).
- The establishment of insurance arrangements for catastrophic diseases. Industrial sectors (e.g. mining and railways) in some cities set up insurance schemes for catastrophic disease for their employees and retirees in order to increase risk-pooling capacity and scale. This initiative was mainly developed in the LIS.
- The use of capitation in the management of the GIS. Some municipal governments gave designated hospitals the GIS fund as annual capitation payments. These hospitals were then expected to provide defined services to the beneficiaries. Usually these hospitals had to share some financial risks if they overspent the funds allocated to them. However, if they spent less than the amount budgeted, they were allowed to keep a portion of the savings for hospital development.

It is difficult to assess the reforms undertaken in this period, since there was almost no scientific research done in this area and health economics was a very new subject until the late 1980s. One of the main actions taken was the introduction of co-payment mechanisms, which was the only action to tackle the problems associated with demand-side behaviour. On the whole, few reforms attempted to influence the behaviour of service providers. In addition, this uneven approach may have reduced the demand for services in general and not just those that were unnecessary. Cost-recovery mechanisms such as co-payments[5] can also have the effect of reducing access to non-acute/preventive care. This leads to an initial drop in costs which is not necessarily cost-effective in the long term.

Phase Two began in 1988 when the central government assumed a leading role by establishing a group to guide the reform of urban employee health insurance schemes. This group was headed by the Ministry of Health, but it also involved nine ministries including Finance, Personnel and Labour. A draft document entitled 'Considerations on the Reform of the Employee Health Insurance System' was issued in July 1988, setting out the direction for reforming the GIS and LIS. An experimental reform of the GIS and LIS commenced in the four cities of Dandong, Siping, Huangshi and Zhuzhou in early 1989.

The main purpose of these experiments was to establish city-wide health insurance systems with the introduction of some cost-control mechanisms. Unfortunately, the systems in the four cities were not developed as expected, owing to a lack of interest on the part of local governments and the fiscal difficulties facing these cities. Only Dandong completed the design of the health insurance scheme. However, Dandong was unable to implement its plan.[6]

In 1992 the leading group for reforming the GIS and LIS was upgraded. It was directed by a State Councillor and was under the direct leadership of the State Council. Its main purpose during Phase Two was to guide the reform of the GIS and LIS in two demonstration cities (Zhengjiang and Jiujiang), later expanding to 57 cities. In fact, in the early 1990s there were a number of urban health insurance reform experiments initiated in other cities and provinces, such as Hainan, Shenzhen and Shanghai, with support from central government. However, the experiment in Zhengjiang and Jiujiang played the most important role in shaping the new basic health insurance schemes in urban China in Phase Three.

Zhengjiang and Jiujiang experiment
In 1994 a health insurance reform experiment began in Zhengjiang City in Jiangsu Province and Jiujiang City in Jiangxi Province under the auspices of the State Council. These two cities, each of which has about 2.5 million inhabitants, set out to develop a new model of urban health insurance. Both cities required that every institution which had GIS and LIS should participate.

Newly established health insurance management centres collected insurance premiums from the government agencies, public institutions, and enterprises, then allocated these funds to individual accounts and a pooled social risk fund. The percentage of these funds allocated to individual accounts from the employers' contributions usually depended on the age of the beneficiaries. The financial contribution from the employees' salaries usually went to their own individual accounts. Three tiers of payment were developed using the individual accounts and the social risk fund (see Box 2.1).

Box 2.1 Three tiers of payment for medical care in the Zhengjiang and Jiujiang health insurance experiment

The first tier – All individuals first used their own individual accounts to pay for medical care. Approximately 5–7 per cent of salary was deposited periodically into individual accounts depending on age.

The second tier – Once the insured person had used up the funds in his or her individual account, medical care was paid out of pocket until the payments reached 5 per cent of their annual income.

The third tier – After paying 5 per cent of his or her annual wage/salary out of pocket for medical care, the insured was eligible to use the social risk fund to pay for medical care. However, the new health insurance schemes in both cities required a deductible and co-insurance payment of up to 20 per cent of medical care expenditure at this tier.

The introduction of individual accounts and co-payment mechanisms was expected to encourage moderation in the demand for medical care in the two cities. In addition, the new health insurance schemes also developed an essential drug list consisting of about 1,400 Western pharmaceutical products and about 500 manufactured Chinese medicines. Only the drugs on the list were covered by the schemes in the two cities.

However, due to overspending of the social risk fund in Zhengjiang, the health insurance management committee in 1999 decided that the fund from the individual accounts could only be used to pay for out-patient services, and the social risk fund could mainly be used to pay for in-patient services and special out-patient services for a limited number of chronic diseases (Wang and Wang, 1999). Such an approach has implications for equity in financing of and access to health care, issues that will be discussed later.

After more than one year of experimentation in the two cities, the State Council decided to expand the experiment to 57 cities in 1996, using the same principles, but allowing these cities to modify the model according to their local situation. About 40 of these cities reformed their GIS and LIS. Even among those cities undertaking reform, some modified the GIS but not the LIS. Poor participation in these schemes was largely due to the inability or unwillingness of some enterprises or their managers to join.

It is neither possible nor practical to describe all of these reforms here. However, experiments worth mentioning are those in Shanghai and Beijing. In order to increase the capacity and scope of social pooling, the Shanghai Municipal Government developed the Hospital Insurance Scheme in 1996, which was mainly funded via payments from employers (4.5 per cent of employee wage/salary). In 1997, the contribution from employers increased to 6.5 per cent. In 1995, the Beijing Municipal Government introduced Catastrophic Diseases Insurance. All enterprises were asked to contribute 6 per cent of the average city employees' income into the fund for each of their employees and retirees. Employees contributed 1 per cent of their own wage/salary into the fund, which was mainly used to cover in-patient services.[7]

Basic health insurance schemes
Phase Three began with the arrival of a new government led by Premier Zhu Rongji in 1997. The new government was restructured in a manner consistent with the new socio-economic order in China. One significant change related to urban health insurance was that the Ministry of Labour and Social Security (MOLSS) was established, building upon the old Ministry of Labour. The MOLSS was mandated by the State Council to take charge of the urban health insurance and its reform. The Department of Medical Insurance of the MOLSS was created to oversee the reform of the GIS and LIS.

Drawing on experience gained from the experiments carried out during Phases One and Two, the new ministry in 1998 advocated new plans for reform over a period of three to five years. The new health insurance scheme structures and financial frameworks developed in Phase Two were maintained in Phase Three with some modifications. The scheme aimed at providing: a low level of health benefit (low depth); a high level of population coverage (breadth); and a capacity for variation, so that differing levels and types of health insurance (from basic coverage to sophisticated and supplemental insurance) could be developed. These plans were incorporated into an official State Council document (State Council, 1998). In addition, a medical financial assistance programme designed to help the urban poor receive basic health care was also advocated. By offering these options of health care financing, the government hoped to meet the differing constituents' health care needs and expectations.

The basic health insurance schemes (HISs) being developed were designed to be less expensive while providing higher population coverage. Careful consideration was given to programme affordability for local governments, enterprises and individuals. Therefore, employers were asked to contribute 6 per cent of employees' salary for health insurance, instead of 10–11 per cent as in Zhengjiang, Jiujiang and Shanghai, while employees were asked to pay 2 per cent. The low contribution by employers was aimed at enabling most enterprises to participate in the HIS. In addition, private companies and enterprises, joint ventures and the self-employed were also required to participate in the schemes. Table 2.4 compares the main characteristics of the old GIS and LIS with the new basic HIS being established in different cities and municipalities of China. It describes key changes in insurance coverage, financing, risk pooling and cost-sharing mechanisms, as well as use of health services. Some of these changes would have an effect on equity in health care.

In order to help municipal/city governments to design an appropriate health insurance scheme, the MOLSS in June 1999, together with the State Development Planning Commission, the Ministry of Finance, the Ministry of Health and the State Chinese Medicine Management Bureau, issued a proposal on the management of diagnostic and treatment services for a basic HIS to every province and municipality. This proposal mainly set out the rules and guidelines for health services or benefits not covered by the HIS and the kinds of services requiring a co-payment. Using these rules and guidelines, each province and municipality was to develop the scope and list of health services to be fully or partially covered by the new schemes. The essential drug list was developed at the same time (State Council, 1998).

The State Council intentionally gave each province and municipality autonomy over the allocation of collected health insurance funds into individual accounts and social risk funds, the level of deductible payment, and the ceiling and percentage of co-insurance payment, although some guidelines were given (e.g. the co-insurance ceiling should be set at around four times the annual income of an average city employee). As a whole, the State Council sought to ensure that each province and municipality would be able to develop a basic HIS appropriate and acceptable to its local socio-economic development and political environment.

Table 2.4 A comparison of the GIS and LIS with the new HIS in urban China

	GIS and LIS	New HIS
Insurance coverage	Employees and retirees fully covered. Dependants partially covered by LIS.	Employees and retirees only.
Financing	From employers only.	From both employers and employees.
Risk pooling	Self-insured by each individual institution.	Risk pooling at a municipal/city level.
Cost sharing	Almost free medical care for beneficiaries.	Co-payment and ceiling level as well as other cost control measures.
Use of health services	No restrictions.	Essential drug list developed. Other health benefits defined by different schemes.

The allocation of the health insurance fund to the individual accounts and the social risk fund is not complex and mainly uses methods tested in the Zhengjiang and Jiujiang experiment. A common rule is that the individual contribution goes to the individual account, while the employer's contribution is split between the individual account and the social risk fund (subject to age). Recently, however, the use of individual accounts and the social risk fund has become more complicated (Table 2.5). Each municipal government with a basic HIS has developed lengthy regulations on the use of individual accounts and social risk funds.

In short, the new HISs which have been developed in cities have adopted in principle a similar model in terms of financial contributions, population coverage, health benefit arrangements and the use of insurance funds, although there are some variations in the level of financial contributions by employers and the use of funds from individual accounts and social risk fund to pay for out-patient and in-patient services.

Table 2.5 Policies and regulations on the use of funds

Service	Individual account	Social risk fund
Out-patient and emergency services	Eligible.	Eligible in some cities under certain conditions.
Special treatments at out-patient department	Eligible.	Eligible in some cities under certain conditions.
In-patient services	Eligible in some cities.	Eligible, but deductible, co-insurance and ceiling arrangements made.

All these new schemes implemented in hundreds of Chinese cities are aimed at targeting mainly employees and retirees from government agencies, public sector institutions, SOEs and COEs, joint ventures and private firms. They exclude children and adults who are unemployed, largely because there has been no consensus about who should make a financial contribution for them.

In addition, as shown above, the new basic HISs with individual accounts and social risk funds are contributed to jointly by employers and employees. This means that the higher one's salary, the greater the contribution into one's individual account. This could put the less well paid in a disadvantageous position (e.g. less money paid into their individual accounts, but the same percentage of co-payment required). In other words, the introduction of individual accounts by the new HISs has affected many in their decision on the use of type and amount of services. As reported by Gao *et al.* (2001), fewer people, including those covered by basic health insurance schemes, visited health service providers and more people bought drugs from pharmacies themselves. This was mainly because people wanted to spend less money out of pocket or to save the money in their individual accounts.

In their evaluation of the Zhengjiang health insurance experiment, Liu *et al.* (2002) found that the experiment appeared to have a positive impact on improving access and equality of care. For instance, their analysis of the data collected from a multi-year survey indicated that, after the reform, more people obtained care of various types, indicating improved access among the general public after the reform, while among those who accessed care the quantity of care was reduced, suggesting a more equal distribution of care among the general population.

The new HISs have also had an impact on cost containment and economic efficiency. The traditional GIS and LIS provided almost free health services to their beneficiaries who had no incentive to economize on the use of health services. Since the implementation of individual accounts and social risk funds and the adoption of deductible and co-insurance arrangements, the insured have begun to rationalize the use of health services. In addition, different payment methods (e.g. fixed fees for services) introduced by some schemes for paying hospitals for providing services give hospitals different incentives. Hospitals and other health facilities in China have swiftly responded to new provider payment methods. For example, in cities where a fixed payment for out-patient visits was used by the service purchasers to pay service providers, patients were often asked to return to see doctors shortly after their first visit. To achieve this, patients were sometimes given drugs for only two or three days to ensure they made the next visit. As a result, the average number of out-patient visits per person rose significantly, but the quality of service may have been compromised. However, competition among different service providers, which was introduced by the new schemes in some cities, did have an impact on service quality and efficiency.

Summary

Over the past half-century the development of China's urban health sector and health insurance schemes has changed dramatically. The network of urban health care systems was well established during the first three decades of the People's Republic, providing a relatively good health service to the vast majority of the urban population. The two work-related medical insurance schemes developed in the early 1950s played an important role in the improvement of the urban population's health from the 1950s to the 1970s, although the Great Cultural Revolution did negatively affect the development of urban health sector. The economic reform launched in the late 1970s has brought profound changes to urban health care and health insurance schemes. The health sector, like other sectors, has tried to adapt to the transformation of China's economy from a planned economy to a market-oriented one. Revenue from service provision and drugs sale has become the most important source of income for hospitals and probably also for other preventive service institutions. The reform of work-related health insurance schemes tried to rationalize the use of health services and control a rapid rise in medical care costs by introducing many mechanisms targeting service users and providers.

All these changes that have taken place over the past two decades have had great implications for both provision and use of health care services in urban China. While the efficiency of service provision and equity in the financing of health care may have been improved in some aspects, there have still been many problems in developing a more equitable and efficient health care system in urban China.

Notes

1 Personal communication between Shenglan Tang and Prof. Xingyuan Gu in October 2003.
2 The prefecture level was replaced by municipal level in the 1990s in China.
3 There were a few private hospitals operating in the early 1950s. However, almost all the private hospitals started to be fully owned by the State in the late 1950s. By the early 1980s there were virtually no private hospitals in China.
4 Gao and his associates reported in their paper that about 13 per cent of the urban population sampled in the national health service survey in 1998, excluding the pupils and the students attending schools, had no jobs and 8 per cent of them had been laid off. However, in 1993 only 11 per cent of the urban population did not have jobs or were

laid off (Gao *et al.*, 2001). A report published by UNDP (1999) estimated that the rate of unemployment in 1998 was 7.9–8.3 per cent. The official unemployment rate published by the National Bureau of Statistics and the MOLSS was 3.1 per cent at the end of year 2000.

5   The term 'co-payment' here indicates amounts paid by the insurance beneficiary as a result of co-insurance and deductibles.

6   Personal communication between Shenglan Tang and Renhua Cai of the Ministry of Health, China in 1998.

7   Summarized from the document entitled 'Regulations on Beijing Basic Health Insurance Scheme' issued by Beijing Municipal Government in 1995.

Chapter 3

The Cities, the People and Their Health

Youlong Gong, Qingyue Meng, Wei Wang and Shenglan Tang

This chapter focuses on the people, their health and the environment in which they live. Initially, we will concentrate on the cities themselves, outlining the structure of the economy and the changing patterns of urban employment, and revealing the specific socio-economic conditions affecting health-seeking behaviour. Subsequently, data on the demographic structure of Nantong and Zibo is presented, and we show how this has changed in the last two decades. Finally, we examine the burden of major infectious and non-infectious diseases among the study population.

The Study Cities

Nantong

One of 13 prefectures located in Jiangsu Province, one of the most developed provinces in China, Nantong occupies a territory of 8,001 km². In 1984 Nantong was one of the first of 14 coastal cities selected by the State Council to be involved in international trading and tourism. Nantong comprises two counties, four county-level cities and four districts. The four districts, Chongchuan, Gangzha, Langshan Tourist District and Fumin Harbour Agency, cover 224 km² and constitute the prefecture city or 'downtown Nantong'.[1] It is in this zone that the detailed studies presented in this book took place. The study covered only the urban population living in the centres of the city and towns. It is not easy for outsiders to understand the Chinese administrative system. Traditionally, the urban population lives in towns or centres of the city and was not given a piece of land by the government in the early 1950s to work on, while the rural population usually lives outside towns or centres of the city and was allocated a piece of land to work on after the founding of People's Republic of China.

Twenty years of economic reforms have boosted Nantong's economy and led to a surge in development. In 1978, Nantong's GDP was only CNY362.4 million; by 1996 it had reached CNY6,859.4 million.[2] From 1986 to 1999 in downtown Nantong, GDP increased 7.47 times and per capita GDP 6.21 times: from CNY1,804.31 million in 1986, a per capita GDP of CNY3,415, to CNY15.99 billion in 2000, a per capita GDP of CNY24,619 (Nantong Statistical Yearbook, 2001). Income levels have risen accordingly. In downtown Nantong in 1997, the average annual income of employees was CNY8,032. The highest income, CNY17,749 a year, was derived from joint-venture enterprises, and the lowest, CNY6,241 a year, from COEs (Nantong Statistical Bureau, 2001). The latter figure is still higher than the average yearly income of employees in Chinese cities, which amounted to about CNY4,000 in 1997. Whilst such indicators point to a healthy economy and appear to confirm that a vast majority of businesses and employees in Nantong should be able to support a health insurance premium, the reality is more complex.

Radical reform of the enterprise sector, especially since 1994, has resulted in far-reaching changes which have had different impacts. Multi-ownership systems have been encouraged as a means of developing a production economy in place of the original predominantly publicly owned economic system. A breakdown of 2,053 businesses in Nantong in 1997 revealed: 636 public and government institutions; 404 state-owned enterprises/factories and companies/firms; 575 collectively owned enterprises/factories and companies/firms; 15 joint-venture; 196 stock-shared; 133 foreign-backed; 80 supported by Hong Kong, Taiwan and Macau; and 14 others (Nantong Statistical Bureau, 1998). In the last two decades large and middle-scale enterprises have thrived. Non-publicly owned economic forms in particular have mushroomed, their product value in Nantong rising from a little over 0 per cent of total products to 36.6 per cent from 1978 to 1997 (Nantong Statistical Bureau, 1998).

However, many middle- and small-scale enterprises, principally SOEs and COEs, have encountered difficulties, operating in minor profit or at a loss. The product value of SOEs from 1978 to 1997 declined from 59.9 per cent to just 16.5 per cent of total products (Nantong Statistical Bureau, 1998).[3] This has occurred because of reform of the state enterprise sector. State subsidies have been withdrawn and radical measures have been implemented such as labour force reduction and the closure of non-profit-making businesses. Predictably, bankrupt SOEs and the numbers of laid-off workers have increased.

Zibo

Zibo is one of 17 prefectures in Shandong Province, the second most populated province, and occupies an area of 5,900 km². Zibo is organized into three counties, Huantai, Yiyuan and Gaoqing, and five districts: Zhangdian, Zhoucun, Boshan, Zichuan and Linzi. In 1999, there were 120 townships/towns under the eight districts and counties and 3,500 villages within the townships/towns. Unlike other prefectures, the central city is scattered; Zibo is actually composed of five satellite cities.

In 1980 Zibo's GDP was CNY26.01 billion, a per capita GDP of CNY768. By 1999 GDP had reached CNY56.8 billion, a per capita GDP of CNY14,035. The yearly growth rate of government income from 1985 to 1999, principally from industrial and commercial taxes and enterprise income tax, was about 11.26 per cent. The majority of enterprises are very small and located at the village level. In 1997 only 986 (6.25 per cent) out of 15,776 enterprises were at or above township level. Of these, 103 were state-owned; 431 collectively owned; 122 privately owned; 215 share-holding; 113 joint ventures; plus 2 others, which are located at the district/county, township and village levels.

In Zibo pressure for enterprise reform has been intense because textile production and heavy industry are the major components of its economy. The industrial and commercial sector employs 56.7 per cent of total urban employees. In 1999 20 per cent of enterprises were officially declared bankrupt. However, in the past few years it has been estimated that about 40 per cent of enterprises in Zibo have been at or approaching bankruptcy, 40 per cent have broken even, and only 20 per cent have been able to make a profit. In 1997 the official reported unemployment rate in the urban area was 2.1 per cent and by 1999 450,000 people were registered unemployed; however, the actual number is purportedly at least five times higher, according to one deputy director of the Municipal Bureau of Labour and Social Security in Zibo. In addition, there is no official statistical information on the number of temporarily unemployed workers. If one measures the total available labour force in urban areas against the number of employees, it becomes clear that about 40 per cent of productive people have no formal jobs. An income support scheme, as part of the establishment of a comprehensive social security system for unemployed and laid-off workers, was created at the end of 2000 to help those who lost their jobs. In 1999 there were 97,070 self-employed workers, accounting for 18.5 per cent of total urban employees. This number will increase as enterprise reforms are being implemented.

Demographic Structure

In order to understand the data on the demographic structure of Nantong and Zibo it is important to take into account the impact of the system of household registration on the measurement of the urban and rural population. As described in Chapter 1, households have been registered as either urban or rural since the 1950s and they have not been allowed to move without official permission. Since the late 1970s an increasing number of people have moved from urban to rural areas. In theory, these temporary migrants are expected to register with the police; in practice, many do not. Consequently, the official data on the numbers of migrants may be underestimates. The precise number of this 'floating' population is uncertain, but is thought to be at least double official estimates. This population is not covered by any social insurance system. Whether they have any insurance status at all is determined solely by their employer, if they have been fortunate enough to secure a job. In fact it is extremely difficult for rural-to-urban migrants to find permanent jobs in cities, because most jobs offered by SOEs or COEs or public and government institutions are reserved for officially registered urban residents or those who have obtained university degrees.

There are plans in the near future to completely overhaul the household registration system in China. In some large cities, the dual systems of urban and rural registration have gradually been phased out. In Guangdong, for instance, the boundary between rural and urban residents has been removed. People can relocate anywhere within the province and are eligible for social insurance benefits regardless of their original place of residence. Jiangsu Province, where Nantong is located, has also started to reform the registration *hukou* system, giving people who do not have an official resident status in its cities a right to work. This reform has provided an environment that is highly conducive to the free movement of people, a prerequisite of a market-oriented economy, and, importantly, gives rural-to-urban migrants vital welfare protection.

Nantong

In 1985 the total population of Nantong was 7.45 million. Owing principally to the effective implementation of the 'one child, one family' policy, by 1998 that figure had risen only slightly to 7.88 million, and by 1999 had dropped back a tiny amount to 7.86 million. However, the urban population rose rapidly between 1985 and 2000: from 1.52 million in 1985 to 3.78 million by 2000 (Nantong Statistical Bureau, 2001) (see Table 3.1). However, the precise number of the urban population is uncertain owing to the altering of boundaries between urban and rural areas. In other words, the proportion of the people in Nantong regarded as urban population rose from 20.4 per cent in 1985 to 48.2 per cent. By 1999, downtown Nantong had a population of 0.64 million (Nantong Social and Economic Statistics for 1993–9). This rapid increase in urban inhabitants can be attributed partly to the establishment of more cities, particularly county-level cities, and partly to an increase in legal immigrants from rural areas since the mid-1980s. As a whole, the progress of the urbanization in this eastern coastal city has been significant over the past two decades.

Table 3.1 Population numbers (millions) in Nantong in selected years

	1985	1990	1995	2000
Urban population	1.52	1.53	2.12	2.53
Rural population	5.93	6.23	5.72	5.32
Total population	7.45	7.76	7.84	7.85

In 2000, of Nantong's total population 8.2 per cent were over 65 years of age, only 3.8 per cent were children under five and 28.1 per cent were women of childbearing age (15–49 years old). In the same year an analysis of the population occupying downtown Nantong reveals that 13 per cent were over 60 and 9.1 per cent over 65, indicating that Nantong is an ageing city, 3.6 per cent were under five and 30.7 per cent were women of childbearing age. The population ratio of urban male to urban female was about 50.1:49.9, though the proportion of the female population over 60 years old (13.9 per cent) was higher than that of the male population (12.2 per cent).

With regard to the floating population, according to data from police stations, the registered floating population in 1997 was 246,100 in the Nantong downtown area. However, according to Mr Lu, Deputy Director of the Nantong Municipal

Bureau of Labour and Social Security, the actual number was likely to be much higher than the reported one.

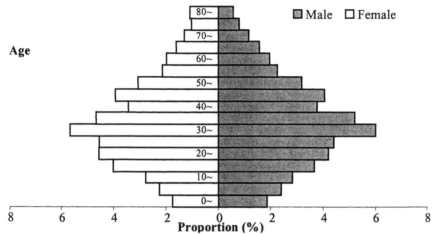

Figure 3.1 Structure of the Nantong population by sex and age, 2000
Source: The Fifth National Census data from Nantong Statistical Bureau.

Zibo

In Zibo, although the natural increase rate of population has declined since 1980, the number of urban residents has mushroomed. In 1980, 19.4 per cent, or 0.66 million, of a total population of 3.4 million resided in urban areas. By 2000, this figure had leapt to 32.9 per cent, that is, 1.37 million of a total population of 4.16 million (Table 3.2). This significant increase is attributable to the change in administrative structure, which came about as part of the urbanization of the city, as well as to population movements within and outside Zibo together with changes in business labour policies. One thing shown in Table 3.2 is that the number of people regarded as rural population has been stable in Zibo since the mid-1980s.

Table 3.2 Population numbers (millions) in Zibo in selected years

	1980	1985	1990	1995	2000
Urban population	0.66	0.84	0.99	1.22	1.37
Rural population	2.48	2.74	2.82	2.72	2.79
Total population	3.14	3.58	3.81	3.94	4.16

Source: Zibo Statistical Yearbook (1980–95); The 2000 Population Census of Shandong Province, China Statistics Press (2002).

Of the urban population of Zibo City, 11.75 per cent were over 60 years old, according to the 2000 National Census data. The proportion of the female population over 60 years old (13.23 per cent) was much higher than that of the male population (10.27 per cent). Nearly one-fifth of the urban population in the city was under 15 years of age in 2000. The population ratio of urban male to urban female was almost 50:50 in 2000.

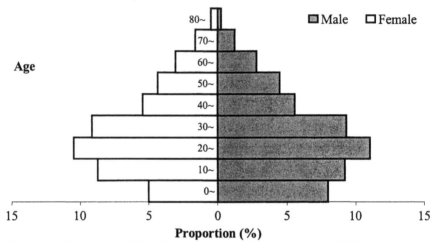

Figure 3.2 Structure of the Zibo population by sex and age, 2000
Source: The Fifth National Census data from Shandong Statistical Bureau (2002).

With regard to the floating population, according to official data, there were 146,018 people originally resident outside the cities living in urban areas in 1995. However, as stated before, deficiencies in the registration system mean that one can realistically double the official figure. The yearly increase rate of this population group was estimated by local officials to be about 15–20 per cent. For the reasons discussed above, it is formidably difficult to get accurate figures of how many of the floating population are living in the urban areas of Zibo unless a population census is conducted.

Health Indices

Nantong

The birth rate, infant mortality rate (IMR) and maternal mortality rate (MMR) are all lower than the national average in Nantong. The birth rate in the whole of Nantong rose from 9.66 per 1,000 population in 1985 to 16.40 per 1,000 in 1989, and in urban areas it increased from 8.61 per 1,000 population in 1985 to 14.60 per 1,000 in 1989. It then declined to the level of around 9 per 1,000 population in the whole of Nantong and in urban areas in the late 1990s.[4] This may imply that, due to rapid development of the local economy and the urbanization of the city, the difference in birth rates between the urban and rural rich areas of China has been closing.

The crude mortality rate, as a whole, increased slightly between 1985 and 1998 in both the total population and in the urban areas (Table 3.3). However, on the whole, the rate has remained at around 7 per 1,000 people for the total population and 5 per 1,000 for the urban population. It is not surprising, therefore, that the rate of population growth rose in the second half of the 1980s and then declined from 9.90 per 1,000 population in 1989 to 1.67 per 1,000 population in 2000 in the whole of Nantong, and in downtown Nantong from 9.30 per 1,000 population in 1989 to 3.74 per 1,000 population in 1998. A possible reason for the difference in urban and rural population growth rates might be a difference in the mortality rates between the two areas. By 1999, the growth rate of the total population of Nantong stood at a level of just 0.35 per 1,000.

Table 3.3 Birth rate, infant mortality rate, mortality rate and natural growth rates of the Nantong population, 1985–2000

Year	Birth rate ‰	IMR ‰	Mortality rate ‰	Natural increase rate ‰
1985	9.66	n/a	6.64	3.02
1986	12.83	11.82	6.74	6.09
1987	15.37	13.44	6.75	8.62
1988	14.90	15.37	6.59	8.31
1989	16.40	17.61	6.50	9.90
1990	14.80	19.30	7.00	7.80
1991	11.24	15.64	6.71	4.53
1992	10.05	15.27	7.11	2.94
1993	10.19	n/a	6.99	3.20
1994	10.17	n/a	7.00	3.17
1995	10.37	n/a	7.17	3.20
1996	9.00	n/a	7.09	1.91
1997	8.68	12.54	6.97	1.71
1998	9.15	12.70	7.53	1.62
1999	7.53	n/a	7.18	0.35
2000	8.80	9.84	7.13	1.67

Source: Nantong Statistical Bureau (2001).

Although the IMR rose between 1986 and 1990, generally speaking it has remained low, declining from 19.3 per 1,000 live births in 1990 to 9.84 per 1,000 live births in 2000. The fluctuation is due most likely to inherent weaknesses in the death reporting system. Instances of this were greatly reduced after 1990 with the implementation of the Primary Health Care (PHC) programme, which strengthened the collection and management of statistical data relating to health. The MMR has varied tremendously, standing at 23.19 per 100,000 live births in 1997, but remaining at zero in many other years because of the low birth rate. With regard to urban/rural variations, the IMR was 37.7 per 1,000 in rural areas and 13.1 per 1,000 in urban areas in 1997, whilst the MMR was 80.4 per 100,000 in rural and 38.3 per 100,000 in urban areas.

The IMR, U5MR (under-five mortality rate) and MMR from 1990 to 2000 for downtown Nantong are presented in Table 3.4. The three mortality rates are quite low in the downtown area. Some of the indicators are much lower than the indicators reported by Shanghai and Beijing. It is difficult to assess the degree to which this reflects real differences in mortality and the degree to which it is due to problems with death notification in Nantong. The authors of the report believe that the IMR, U5MR and MMR in the city are far better than the national averages.

Table 3.4 IMR, U5MR and MMR in downtown Nantong, 1990–2000

Year	IMR(‰)	U5MR(‰)	MMR(1/100,000)
1990	6.42	n/a	21.82
1991	7.62	n/a	23.44
1992	12.94	15.91	21.21
1993	15.60	18.23	20.26
1994	8.38	9.94	0
1995	9.36	11.08	0
1996	10.70	13.91	0
1997	10.21	12.52	23.19
1998	10.02	12.70	0
1999	9.02	n/a	0
2000	6.88	n/a	21.27

Source: Nantong Health Bureau.

Zibo

From 1985 to 2000, the birth rate first declined from 15.75 per 1,000 population in 1986–90 to 11.28 per 1,000 population in 1991–5, and then rose slightly to 12.36 per 1,000 population in 1996–2000. There was no significant change in crude mortality rates (around 5.8 per 1,000 population) over the period. Hence, the population growth rates over the period followed the pattern of birth rates (Table 3.5.).

Table 3.5 Birth, mortality and natural growth rates of the Zibo population, 1985–2000

Years	Birth rate ‰	Mortality rate ‰	Natural growth rate ‰
1986–90	15.75	5.80	10.0
1991–5	11.28	5.82	5.45
1996–2000	12.36	5.82	6.54

Source: Zibo Statistical Yearbook (2001).

It is difficult to explain why the population growth rates were so low in 1991–5. One possibility is that birth rates were under-reported during these years. Another possibility may be the timing of the peak of population growth.[5] The officially reported IMR and MMR in 1997 were, respectively, 12.41 per 1,000 live births and

37.06 per 100,000. There is a great possibility of under-reporting of the two rates in the city, although it is difficult to estimate the extent to which this occurred.

Epidemiological Profile

Nantong

According to a national survey in 1992, the three most common causes of death in the total population of Nantong in the period 1988–91 were malignant tumour, respiratory system diseases and cerebro-vascular diseases. The mortality rates were, respectively, 137.8, 102.3 and 100.5 per 100,000 population in downtown Nantong. Approximately one-quarter of the deaths were associated with cancers, one-fifth with respiratory diseases and another one-fifth with cerebro-vascular diseases. These three diseases accounted for 68.01 per cent of deaths among the total population and 63.61 per cent in downtown Nantong. The fourth and fifth most common causes of death amongst the total population were trauma and toxicosis and heart diseases; these rankings were reversed in downtown Nantong. The five leading diseases accounted for 83.57 per cent of deaths amongst the total population and 80.13 per cent of deaths in downtown Nantong (see Table 3.6).

Table 3.6 The five leading causes of death in Nantong, 1988–91

Rank	Total population			Downtown area		
	Diseases	Proportion %	Mortality (1/100,000)	Diseases	Proportion %	Mortality (1/100,000)
1	Cancer	27.48	185.33	Cancer	25.73	137.82
2	Respiratory system diseases	26.19	176.66	Respiratory system diseases	19.11	102.34
3	Cerebro-vascular diseases	14.34	96.71	Cerebro-vascular diseases	18.77	100.54
4	Trauma and toxicosis	8.16	55.01	Heart diseases	8.64	46.26
5	Heart diseases	7.40	49.89	Trauma and toxicosis	7.88	42.22

Source: Nantong Anti-Epidemic Station.

Table 3.7 shows the ten leading causes of death in Nantong in 1999, sub-divided by gender. The first five are identical to the 1988–91 pattern for the downtown area. Nine of the causes of death are due to non-communicable chronic diseases (NCD), but infectious disease still ranks at number seven. The Nantong City AES refused to provide any information on incidence rates of notifiable infectious diseases, but according to the literature we reviewed, it seems that they have declined significantly since the foundation of the People's Republic. However, the incident rate of hepatitis (particularly Hepatitis A) and diarrhoea had risen remarkably, from 13 per 100,000 population in the 1950s to 465 per 100,000 population in the 1980s, and from 54 per 100,000 population in the 1960s to 235 per 100,000 population in the 1980s. Over the past decade, the incident rates of two infectious diseases have come down slightly (Chen *et al.*, 1998). Table 3.7 reveals that mental illness is prevalent, especially amongst women. Average life expectancy is 75.30 for men and 78.30 for women.

Table 3.7 The ten leading causes of death by sex composition in Nantong, 1999

Rank	Male	Female	Total
1	Malignant tumour	Respiratory system diseases	Malignant tumour
2	Respiratory system diseases	Malignant tumour	Respiratory system diseases
3	Cerebro-vascular diseases	Cerebro-vascular diseases	Cerebro-vascular diseases
4	Heart diseases	Trauma and toxicosis	Heart diseases
5	Trauma and toxicosis	Heart diseases	Trauma and toxicosis
6	Digestive system diseases	Digestive system diseases	Digestive system diseases
7	Infectious diseases	Mental diseases	Infectious diseases
8	Neonatal diseases	Infectious diseases	Mental diseases
9	Urinary system	Neonatal diseases	Neonatal diseases
10	Mental diseases	Endocrine and immunology	Urinary system

Source: Nantong Statistical Yearbook (2000).

Table 3.8 shows the disease classification in eight urban general hospitals (including county-level cities) in Nantong in 1998. In a departure from the death pattern, digestive system disease ranks number one, trauma and toxicosis rank second and have the highest total admission days, and pregnancy, childbirth and puerperium complications rank third. Interestingly, hospitalizations due to injury rose from 7,806 cases in 1995 to 11,104 cases in 1999, becoming the primary cause of hospitalization in 1999. This may imply rising problems related to traffic and workplace accidents, which could be seen as a result of rapid economic development that has not been well regulated and managed.

It is evident that, although the death pattern in Nantong is due predominantly to non-communicable chronic diseases, acute and infectious diseases are still important causes of people's ill-health. Clearly, the chief priority of the health care system must be to strengthen disease prevention efforts, particularly in controlling the incidence of infectious diseases, especially intestinal infectious disease such as viral hepatitis and dysentery. For example, up to one in seven of the Chinese population is affected by the Hepatitis B virus. In addition, the incidence rate of STDs has been increasing greatly over the past two decades. Regrettably, the fact that health care costs dissuade many of the vulnerable from seeking early diagnosis and treatment for ill-health ultimately creates conditions in which infectious diseases, such as STD and tuberculosis, are more likely to spread.

Table 3.8 Disease classification of in-patients in eight urban hospitals in Nantong, 1998

Rank	Classification of diseases	Number of patients	%	Total bed-days	%
1	Digestive system	10,493	15.07	124,385	13.19
2	Trauma and toxicosis	10,218	14.68	146,770	15.56
3	Pregnancy, childbirth, puerperium complications	9,968	14.32	66,380	7.04
4	Respiratory system	8,756	12.58	107,882	11.44
5	Tumour	7,430	10.67	146,295	15.51
6	Circulatory system	5,912	8.49	124,831	13.24
7	Urinary and reproductive system	3,764	5.41	56,163	5.96
8	Neuro-system	2,644	3.80	36,788	3.90
9	Infectious and parasitic	2,209	3.17	45,832	4.86
10	Muscular, skeleton and connective tissue	1,401	2.01	22,721	2.41
11	Derivation from perinatal period	1,013	1.46	8,928	0.95
12	Endocrine, nutrition, metabolism and immunology	881	1.27	20,861	2.21
13	Congenital abnormality	734	1.05	9,552	1.01
14	Blood and hemopoiesis system	710	1.02	12,143	1.29
15	Diagnosis unclear	632	0.91	6,433	0.68
16	Dermatosis and hypoderm disease	429	0.62	5,821	0.62
17	Mental disorder	96	0.14	1,321	0.14
18	Others	2,324	3.34	0	0.00
	Total	69,614	100.00	943,106	100.00

Source: Nantong Health Bureau.

Zibo

In Zibo City in 2000 the first three most common causes of death were malignant tumours, cerebro-vascular diseases and heart diseases, accounting for 23.9 per cent, 21.6 per cent and 16.8 per cent of deaths (62.3 per cent of the total). The fourth and fifth leading causes were respiratory system diseases and trauma and toxicosis (Table 3.9).

Table 3.9 The ten leading causes of death in Zibo, 2000

Cause of death	%
Total	**91.96**
1 Malignant tumour	23.89
2 Cerebro-vascular disease	21.63
3 Heart disease	16.82
4 Respiratory system disease	13.89
5 Trauma and toxicosis	6.28
6 Digestive system disease	3.04
7 Internal system, nutrition, metabolism and immune system disease	2.87
8 Urinary system disease	1.51
9 Mental disease	1.13
10 Neuropathy	0.90
Male	**92.67**
1 Malignant tumour	26.70
2 Cerebro-vascular disease	21.11
3 Heart disease	15.61
4 Respiratory system disease	13.47
5 Trauma and toxicosis	7.02
6 Digestive system disease	3.32
7 Internal system, nutrition, metabolism and immune system disease	2.12
8 Urinary system disease	1.42
9 Mental disease	0.98
10 Neuropathy	0.92
Female	**91.03**
1 Malignant tumour	22.25
2 Cerebro-vascular disease	20.42
3 Heart disease	18.31
4 Respiratory system disease	14.40
5 Trauma and toxicosis	5.37
6 Digestive system disease	3.79
7 Internal system, nutrition, metabolism and immune system disease	2.68
8 Urinary system disease	1.62
9 Mental disease	1.32
10 Neuropathy	0.87

Source: Zibo Health Statistics (2001).

Most infectious diseases are notifiable diseases, according to the infectious disease prevention and treatment law passed by the People's Congress of the People's Republic of China. However, the implementation of this policy has not been effective in many places of China. Hence, the incident rate of many infectious diseases, based on the notification data, was under-reported. The data of notifiable infectious diseases from Zibo show that the number of infectious diseases declined from 17,613 cases in 1985 to 6,591 in 1995, and then rose slightly to 9,319 cases in 1997. However, the mortality rate rose from 77 per 100,000 population in 1985 to

86 per 100,000 population in 1990, and then declined significantly to 38 and 33 per 100,000 population in 1995 and 1997.

Dysenteric diarrhoea was the most common infectious disease in Zibo. The incidence rate increased from 67.8 per 100,000 population in 1994 to 108.2 per 100,000 population in 1997. The next most common infectious diseases were hepatitis and meningitis. Tuberculosis was not listed as one of the top ten infectious diseases before 1997. However, in 1997 it jumped to third place in Zibo City with a reported incidence rate of 23 per 100,000 population, according to the notification data.

Notes

1 Chongchuan and Gangzha are original districts and Langshan Tourist District and Fumin Harbour Agency were newly created in the 1990s.
2 Nantong's GDP here included the GDP of downtown Nantong (i.e. the four districts listed and the GDP of two counties and four county-level cities administrated by the Nantong Municipal Government).
3 The term 'product value' was derived from the planned economy in which the enterprises sold their products to the state with the prices defined by the government. The product value indicates the total amount of money that can theoretically be generated from the sale of their products.
4 The Department of Police reports this data to the Department of Statistics. Thus, government agencies can obtain population information from either department.
5 The first peak of population growth in China was in the early 1950s and the second one was in the mid-1960s. The period between 1985 and 1989 was the time when those born in the 1960s were expected to get married and have children. Therefore, the population growth in the late 1980s was called the third peak of population growth.

Chapter 4

The Health Systems of Nantong and Zibo

Qingyue Meng, Zhonghua Weng, Ning Zhuang, Wei Wang, Qiang Sun, Yuelai Lu, Baogang Shu and Gerald Bloom

This chapter introduces the health systems of Nantong and Zibo. It describes the structure of their health services, presents some descriptive data, looks at health finance and expenditure and concludes with a discussion of health reform in the two cities.

Organization of the Health Sector

The government is organized into national, provincial, municipal, county (rural) or district (urban) and township (rural) or street (urban) levels. It is also organized in vertical structures that extend from the national level to the lowest level. The two city governments have similar structures. To avoid repetition this chapter presents diagrams describing one city and points out differences between the two.

Both cities have a municipal health bureau, which is responsible for health services throughout the city and for municipal-level health facilities (Figure 4.1). They have a number of county (rural) or district (urban) health bureaux, which answer to county or district governments. They also have township and community health centres, which relate to local administrative structures. The township or community health centres were previously under the administrative control of the lowest level of government, but a recent government policy has put them under county or district governments.

A number of departments of the Nantong and Zibo governments have health-related responsibilities. The Bureau of Health is responsible for policy-making, health service provision and health care regulation and it administers all government health facilities. Labour and Social Security has primary responsibility for managing and implementing the urban health insurance scheme. Finance allocates public sector budgets and Planning is responsible for the formulation and implementation of development plans. Family Planning oversees a network of facilities that provide family planning services. Civil Affairs formulates policies of assistance to vulnerable groups, including the provision of subsidized health services.

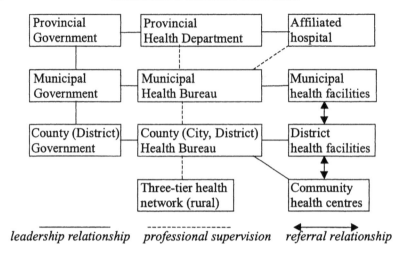

leadership relationship   professional supervision   referral relationship

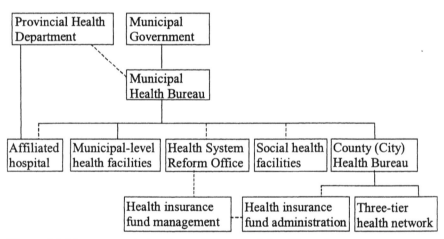

Figure 4.1 Management structure of Nantong's health system

The division of responsibilities between so many agencies has made it difficult to formulate and implement comprehensive health development strategies. The reason for this is illustrated in Figure 4.2, which shows that each of Zibo's three Deputy Mayors have oversight of at least one bureau with a major health responsibility. This creates formidable problems of coordination. Nantong has tried to address this problem by creating a Municipal Health System Reform Steering Group on which all relevant departments are represented (Figure 4.1). One of its major responsibilities is to liaise with the institutions responsible for health insurance reform.

Both Municipal Health Bureaux supervise the district- and county-level health bureaux and directly manage municipal-level health facilities (Figure 4.1).

Nantong Municipality also partly manages the affiliated hospital of Nantong Medical College, in accordance with directives of the Jiangsu Provincial Health Department and the Nantong Municipal Government. Both Health Bureaux have similar structures. Nantong's is organized into divisions of: General Administration; Medical Administration; Pharmaceuticals; Disease Control and Prevention (formerly Anti-Epidemic Services); Primary Health and Maternal and Child Health; Traditional Chinese Medicine; Research and Education; and Personnel.

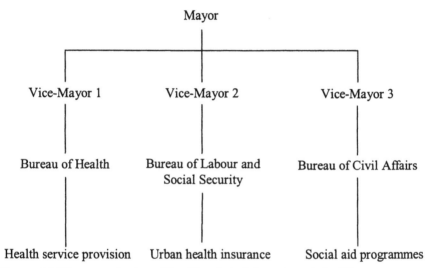

Figure 4.2 The organization of health-related departments in Zibo

The hospitals are managed by various administrative agencies. Zibo's Municipal Hospital is directly managed by the Municipal Health Bureau. County and district hospitals are managed by county or district health bureaux. Township and community health centres have been managed by the equivalent level of government but, according to a recent national policy statement, they will be managed by the county or district level in future. Health facilities outside the health sector, for example military hospitals or clinics or hospitals in business enterprises, are administered by their own governing bodies, with technical overview by the Health Bureau.

Health Services

Preventive Programmes

The preventive services are organized largely by the Centre for Disease Control and Prevention (CDC) and the Maternal and Child Health (MCH) centres. Nantong also has an STD Surveillance Centre. The CDC is responsible for disease control and prevention, including immunization programmes, surveillance for infectious diseases and environmental health. The MCH Centre oversees maternal and child health care. In Nantong the STD Surveillance Centre records and examines STD epidemics and provides health education. At municipal and county (district) level, these facilities operate independently under the administrative authority of the Health Bureaux. In townships, preventive programmes are implemented by specific groups within township health centres.

Facilities

Both cities have a network of health facilities belonging to different levels of government and different government or private agencies. Nantong has 303 hospitals and township health centres (THC), of which 10 are run by non-health institutions and enterprises (Table 4.1). The government classifies in-patient facilities into three grades based on the facility, equipment and staffing. The higher the grade, the more sophisticated the facility. Nantong has 3 grade III hospitals, all located in the city centre; it has 20 grade II hospitals, of which 3 are in the downtown area; and there are 284 grade I hospitals, of which 13 are in the downtown area. Zibo has 132 hospitals and health centres, of which 124 are managed by the health authorities (Table 4.2). The rest are owned and run by enterprises and the military.

Table 4.1 Health facilities in Nantong, 2000

Category	Total	Health sector	Other sectors
Hospitals and health centres	303	292	11
Municipal level	9	9	–
County/district level	33	22	11
Township/community health centres	261	261	–
Other facilities			
Sanatoriums	1	–	1
Clinics	760	19	741
Special disease control centres	10	9	1
Health and anti-epidemic stations	10	9	1
MCH centres	7	7	–
Other health facilities	25	21	4
Privately run clinics	739	–	739
Village clinics*	3,676	–	–

* Many village clinics are owned and run by the village collectives. Some township health centres are public institutions but others are collectively owned.
Source: Nantong Health Bureau.

Table 4.2 Health facilities in Zibo, 2000

Category	Total	Health sector	Other sectors
Hospitals	132	124	8
Municipal level	3	2	1
District and county level	23	16	7
Township health centres	106	106	–
Other facilities			
Clinics	436	230	206
Health and anti-epidemic stations	9	9	–
MCH centres	9	9	–
Village clinics	3,103	3,103	–

Nantong's hospitals and health centres have 18,747 beds and employ 27,653 people, of whom 21,767 are trained health workers (Table 4.3). Only 3,646 beds are located in urban areas. Other facilities employ 5,583 people. There are also 6,845 village health workers. Zibo's hospitals and health centres have 13,953 beds and employ 17,277 people, of whom 13,660 are trained health workers (Table 4.4). Other facilities employ 4,843 people. Data on village health workers were not available for Zibo.

Data are not usually kept on the allocation of facilities, personnel and budgets between urban and rural localities within the city boundaries. However, the entitlements of urban and rural dwellers are quite different. It is very difficult for city officials to get a clear picture of the relative needs of urban and rural people and of the differences in the health services provided for them.

Table 4.3 In-patient beds and staff of health institutions in Nantong, 2000

Facilities	Beds	Total employees	Trained health workers
Hospitals and health centres	18,747	27,653	21,764
Municipal level	3,601	5,133	3,751
District level	611	696	534
County level	7,924	12,280	9,598
Township health centres	6,611	9,544	7,881
Other facilities			
Sanatoriums	150	46	18
Clinics	0	1,875	1,870
Special disease control centres	350	232	156
AESs	12	742	527
MCH centres	0	217	164
Other health service facilities	527	1,732	828
Privately run clinics	0	739	739
Village clinics	0	6,845	6,845*

* Village health workers are categorized differently from government-employed health workers and not all are trained.
Source: Nantong Health Bureau (2001).

Table 4.4 In-patient beds and staff of health institutions in Zibo, 2000

Facilities	Beds	Total employees	Trained health workers
Hospitals and health centres	13,953	17,277	13,660
Municipal level	11,012	13,372	10,445
County and district	1,213	1,498	1,203
Township health centres	1,728	2,407	2,012
Rehabilitation institutions	129	210	132
Clinics	–	3,118	3,087
AESs	40	1,109	972
MCH centres	75	308	258
Other health service facilities	–	98	45

Source: Zibo Health Statistics (2001).

Health Service Activities

Table 4.5 shows the number of out-patient visits and in-patient admissions in various types of health facility in Nantong in 2000. Township health centres, utilized predominantly by the rural population, are the most important health providers. County general hospitals are the second most important health providers; the majority of their users are rural residents. The municipal hospitals are the primary health providers for the urban population. The occupancy rates for the municipal and county hospitals were relatively high, but the district hospitals and township health centres had very low occupancy rates.

Table 4.5 Utilization of medical services in Nantong, 2000

Category	Out-patient visits	In-patient admission	Occupied bed-days	Bed-days per in-patient	Occupancy rate %
Municipal level	1,602,919	56,124	55,916	18	79
District level	69,028	898	873	18	34
County level	1,738,667	73,909	73,865	15	70
Township health centres	5,889,405	170,529	170,395	7	34

Note: Unable to separate patients' utilization into urban and rural.
Source: Nantong Health Bureau (2001).

There were around 11 million out-patient visits to Zibo's hospitals in 1999 (Table 4.6); 75 per cent of these services were provided by county (district) and municipal-level hospitals (run by government or enterprises). Approximately 267,000 patients were admitted, and around 78 per cent of them were in county (district) and municipal hospitals.

Table 4.6 Utilization of medical services in Zibo, 1999

Health facilities	Number of out-patient visits	Number of hospital admissions
General hospitals	2,400,000	101,000
Chinese traditional hospitals	785,000	20,000
Enterprise hospitals	4,410,000	3,000
Others	505,000	84,000
Township hospitals	2,700,000	59,000
Total	10,800,000	267,000

Source: Zibo Statistical Yearbook (2000).

Health Finance

This section reports the findings of a study on health financing in Nantong undertaken by Baogang Shu, using national accounting methods. The report is supplemented with general information on Zibo.

There are three major sources of health finance in Nantong: government budgets, social risk funds and out-of-pocket payments (Table 4.7). Government health budgets account for a diminishing share of total health expenditure. Their share fell from 16.7 to 13.5 per cent between 1993 and 2000, whilst the share provided by individuals rose from 43.2 to 50.7 per cent. During the same period, total health expenditure rose from CNY818 million to CNY2,670 million (Table 4.8). GDP rose at approximately the same rate so that health expenditure accounted for around 3.3 per cent of GDP throughout this period, substantially lower than the national average of 4.8 per cent in 1998.

Table 4.7 Sources of health finance in Nantong (CNY million), 1993–2000

	1993	1994	1995	1996	1997	1998	1999	2000
Total health expenses	818	983	1,089	1,622	1,788	1,897	2,224	2,670
Budgetary health expenses	137	204	232	239	268	287	319	360
Budgetary health expenses as percentage of total (%)	16.7	20.7	21.3	14.7	15.0	15.2	14.3	13.5
Social health expenses	353	389	428	682	750	802	936	957
Social health expenses as percentage of total (%)	43.2	40.0	39.3	42.1	41.9	42.3	42.1	35.8
Individual health expenses	328	390	429	701	771	808	970	1,353
Individual health expenses as percentage of total (%)	40.1	39.7	39.4	43.2	43.1	42.6	43.6	50.7

Source: Nantong Health Bureau data, Nantong total health expenses table (1993–2000).

Table 4.8 Total health expenses and GDP in Nantong, 1993–9

Year	1993	1994	1995	1996	1997	1998	1999	2000
Total health expenses (million)	818	983	1,089	1,622	1,788	1,897	2,224	2,670
GDP (billion)	25.1	32.8	46.7	54.0	58.0	62.4	67.0	74.3
% of total health expense in GDP	3.26	3.00	2.33	3.00	3.10	3.04	3.32	3.59
Health expenditure per person per year (CNY)	105	126	139	207	228	241	283	340

Source: Nantong Health Bureau data, Nantong total health expenses table (1993–2000).

Health's share of government expenditure fell from 12.6 per cent to 10.5 per cent between 1993 and 1999 (Table 4.9). Government health expenditure includes budgetary allocations to providers of health services and the government insurance scheme (GIS). Between 1993 and 1999, spending on GIS did not rise as quickly as total health budgets (Table 4.10). Expenditure on public health providers rose from CNY10.4 to CNY25.9 per capita.

Table 4.9 Health's share of government budgetary expenditure (CNY million), 1993–9

Year	1993	1994	1995	1996	1997	1998	1999
Government expenditure[a]	1,086	1,459	1,731	2,019	2,389	2,707	3,044
Government health expenditure[b]	137	204	232	239	268	287	319
Health's share of total government expenditure (%)	12.6	14.0	13.4	11.8	11.2	10.6	10.5

Source: [a] Nantong Social and Economic Statistics (1993–9); [b] Nantong Health Bureau data, Nantong total health expenses table (1993–9).

Table 4.10 Government health budgets (CNY million), 1993–9

Year	1993	1994	1995	1996	1997	1998	1999
Budgetary health expenses	137	204	232	239	268	287	319
GIS budget	55	85	105	98	111	112	118
GIS budget as a proportion of total (%)	40.5	41.8	45.3	40.8	41.4	38.8	37.1

Source: Nantong Health Bureau data, Nantong total health expenses table (1993–9).

Around 70 per cent of the public health care budget is allocated to general operations. The remainder goes to traditional Chinese medicine, family planning, medical research, medical education and construction of facilities. Table 4.11 presents data on the allocation of the general operations budget. The proportion allocated to hospitals rose from 23.9 per cent to 31.2 per cent, while the percentage allocated to township health centres stayed relatively constant. The proportion allocated to the AESs and to the MCH centres fell. Nantong allocated only CNY1.3 per person to its AESs and CNY0.4 to its MCH services in 1999.

Table 4.11 Allocation of the general operations budget in Nantong, 1995–9

Year	1995		1997		1998		1999	
	CNY million	%	CNY million	%	CNY million	%	CNY million	%
General operation	90.0	100.0	114.0	100.0	125.0	100.0	120.0	100.0
Hospital expenses	21.5	23.9	29.9	26.2	37.7	30.3	37.4	31.2
Township hospital expenses	31.8	35.2	39.9	35.0	41.0	32.9	43.3	36.1
AES expenses	9.1	10.0	10.3	9.0	10.9	8.8	10.3	8.6
MCH expenses	2.7	2.9	3.4	3.0	3.4	2.7	3.0	2.5
Other expenses	24.9	28.0	30.5	26.8	32.0	25.3	26.0	21.6
AES per capita (CNY)	1.2		1.3		1.4		1.3	
MCH per capita (CNY)	0.3		0.4		0.4		0.4	

Source: Nantong Health Bureau Health Statistics (edited) (1995, 1997–9).

Table 4.12 Hospital income and expenditure (CNY million) in Nantong, 1990 and 2000

Item	Municipal hospitals		County hospitals	
	1990	2000	1990	2000
Total income	52.59	270.59	47.28	360.70
1. Medical service	17.26	117.55	16.44	136.81
2. Pharmacy	30.84	146.51	26.49	214.43
3. Pharmaceutical income	1.57	–	1.50	–
4. Others	2.92	6.53	2.84	9.46
Total expenditure	49.54	287.27	44.80	356.64
1. Service cost	19.40	158.18	17.59	195.95
2. Drugs	29.06	125.59	25.82	154.50
3. Others	1.08	3.50	1.39	6.19
Balance	3.05	–16.68	2.48	4.06
1. Medical service	–2.14	–40.63	–1.15	–59.14
2. Drugs	1.78	20.92	0.67	59.93
3. Others*	3.41	3.03	2.96	3.27
Government complement	4.02	27.95	3.99	23.79
Owed by patients in this year	0.69	–	0.13	–
Surplus after allocation in last year	0	–	0	0.12
Surplus	6.38	10.27	6.34	26.77
Allocation of surplus				
Development fund	2.82	–	3.35	–
Collective welfare fund	1.53	–	0.95	–
Bonus fund	1.85	–	1.74	–
Manager's fund	0.18	–	0.30	–

*Balance is pharmaceutical and other income versus other expenditure.
Source: Nantong Health Bureau (1991 and 2001).

Table 4.12 presents the financial status of Nantong's urban and county hospitals in 1990 and 2000. The urban hospitals include the general hospitals located in the downtown area, and the county hospitals indicate county and county-level city hospitals. In 1990 county-level city hospitals were counted as 'urban', but this was not the case in 2000. That is why the reported income of county hospitals increased so much between the two years. In urban and county hospitals, drug sales account for over half of total revenue and expenditure on drugs takes up more than half of the total expenditure.

Table 4.13 Hospital income and expenditure (CNY10,000) in Zibo, 1990–2000

Items	Municipal hospitals		County hospitals	
	1990	2000	1990	2000
Total income	14,773.1	70,232.4	78,17.4	44,729.9
Medical services	3,163.6	17,851.7	2,072	12,987.8
Out-patient services	1,042.2	6,266.1	603.5	3,989.1
Registration	102.7	430.7	53.8	289.1
Surgical operation	75.8	255.0	29.5	125.2
Examination	772.9	4,829.5	502.9	3,216.1
Others	90.8	750.9	17.3	358.8
In-patient services	2,121.4	11,589.5	1,455.3	8,997.3
Bed fee	540.2	1,704.7	333.4	1,220.2
Surgical operation	110.0	45.3	66.0	500.4
Examination	1,251.2	8,690.9	910.7	6,386.8
Others	220.0	1,148.6	145.2	889.8
Others	18.0	1.6	13.2	1.5
Drugs	6,903.7	32,800.9	3,370.3	20,008.4
Out-patient	4,294.1	20,097.9	1,794.1	11,167.0
In-patient	2,609.6	12,703.0	1,576.2	8,841.3
Government regular budget	1,548.4	6,338.9	609.2	2,370.3
Government specific subsidies	2,683.4	12,635.4	1,574.2	7,516.8
Others	474.0	605.5	191.7	1,846.6
Total expenditures	13,635.0	79,423.8	7,120.2	47,504.7
Salaries	1,251.2	5,686.8	594.6	2,828.3
Social security	260.7	1,246.6	94.9	636.8
Pensions	247.8	12,327.5	72.0	1,193.3
Maintenance	399.6	12,229.2	242.8	1,670.4
Overheads	207.4	12,130.9	112.8	660.9
Utilities	963.5	12,032.6	578.1	4,117.5
Drugs	5,782.3	11,934.2	2,852.8	17,195.8
Medical materials	4,522.5	11,835.9	2,572.2	19,201.7

Source: Zibo Health Department, *Financial Report of Hospitals* (1990 and 2000).

The sources of health finance are similar in Zibo. Owing to a lack of research into health financing in Zibo, the exact composition is not clear. The income and expenditure of Zibo's municipal and county hospitals are listed in Table 4.13. In 2000 38.6 per cent of the revenue of municipal hospitals came from medical services and 50 per cent from the sale of drugs.

In both cities, urban residents have experienced a substantial rise in their out-of-pocket expenditure on health. In 1985 downtown residents of Nantong spent very little on health, since most had work-related health insurance. In 1999 households allocated an average of 4 per cent of annual expenditure to medical care (Nantong Statistical Bureau). In Zibo households spent 0.8 per cent of total expenditure on medical care in 1985; in 1999, health care expenditure claimed 11 per cent of per capita expenditure (*Zibo Statistical Yearbook*, 2000).

Health Insurance

There were two broad categories of urban health insurance scheme until the recent reforms (Table 4.14). The GIS for government employees funded from government budgets, and the LIS for workers in SOEs funded from enterprise welfare funds. The government recommended that COEs provide health insurance, but benefit levels tended to be low. In 1997 Nantong launched a municipal health insurance scheme, which all government institutions and enterprises were invited to join. The schedule for implementing urban health insurance reform in Zibo was set for the end of 2001. All three kinds of insurance scheme persisted throughout the study period. Their characteristics are summarized in Table 4.14.

The government has given high priority to the reform of the system of urban health finance. It began a serious reform effort in the early 1990s with pilot schemes in several medium-sized cities. The first two were in Jiujiang, Jiangxi Province and in Zhenjiang, Jiangsu Province. The schemes were expanded to additional cities, including Nantong. It was found that some units were keen to join, some were reluctant and some joined for only a year or two. Yu and Ren (1998) argue that these responses reflect different interests between enterprises and their employees. The team undertook a survey of enterprises in Nantong to assess whether attitudes to the municipal health insurance scheme were influenced by these factors.

Variations Between Enterprises in the Study Sample

The survey was carried out in December 1999, two and a half years after the launch of the scheme. The sample of 21 units included two government institutions, one public agency, ten SOEs, four COEs and four enterprises of other ownership. The focus groups included managers and medical staff at the sample institutions.

Table 4.14 Characteristics of the major health schemes in Nantong and Zibo

Health scheme	Nantong	Zibo
GIS		
Beneficiaries	Public sector employees. Groups with special entitlements to health benefits (war veterans, senior cadres, etc.).	As for Nantong.
Source of finance	Government health budget.	As for Nantong.
Benefits	Most agencies provide part reimbursement for out- and in-patient services. Medical care is essentially free of charge, except for small registration fees and co-payments. In some profitable agencies or institutions, the reimbursement rate is high, even fully reimbursable. Special groups also have virtually free health care. Industrial injury or work-related illness is treated free of charge.	As for Nantong.
New city-wide municipal insurance scheme		
Beneficiaries	Government agencies and public institutions. Enterprises of their own accord.	Government agencies and public institutions.
Source of finance	Government agency budgets, enterprises and employees.	Government agency budgets and employees.
Benefits	The funding is split into two parts: individual account and risk-sharing fund. Out-patient care is funded from the individual account until this is depleted, then by out-of-pocket payments. Hospital care is funded from social risk-sharing fund with co-payments and a ceiling. The reimbursement rates for in-patient care vary with age. All members pay a fixed amount for every hospitalization, according to the level of hospital, and can then claim for reimbursement. Members of special groups have virtually free care.	The funding is split into two parts: individual account and risk-sharing fund. All expenditures are met from the individual account first. When this is depleted, members pay out of pocket for amounts up to 5% of annual salary, and can then get reimbursement from the risk-sharing fund. Reimbursement rates differ for out-patient and in-patient care and vary with age.
LIS		
Beneficiaries	Employees and pensioners of all SOEs, most COEs and some other enterprises.	As for Nantong.
Finance	Enterprise welfare fund.	As for Nantong.

Reimbursement	Many enterprises adopted some HIS regulations even though they did not join, and established funds with individual and risk-sharing components. Reimbursement is similar to the Zibo HIS, but the rate is higher. Some enterprises established similar insurance schemes for their employees based on the industrial system. Some others are still running traditional schemes, but reimbursement rates are lower. If an enterprise has its own hospital or clinic, reimbursement rates for out- and in-patient services vary depending on use of this facility. All forms of medical care free of charge except for small registration fees and co-payments. Industrial injury or work-related illness treated at no charge. 50% of cost of medical care for immediate family.	Out-patient: many enterprises provide a fixed amount of money for out-patient service. Some profitable enterprises give partial reimbursement. Very few provide full payment. In-patient: most enterprises provide partial reimbursement. The rate varies with profitability and employee's age (or work years). A few special people get full reimbursement. If the enterprise has its own hospital or clinic, reimbursement rates for out- and in-patient services vary depending on use of this facility.

Partial government insurance or labour insurance for dependants

Beneficiaries	Half (H)-GIS: under-18 children of employees. Half (H)-LIS: all pensioners (excluding retirees)	Retired parents, spouse and children of employees covered by GIS or LIS.
Source of finance	Work units and employees.	Work units.
Benefits	H-GIS: 50–80% of all health expenditure, alternately by father's and mother's unit every other year. Some profitable units provide higher rates of reimbursement. H-LIS: most units provide 50% reimbursement for health expenses for out- and in-patient services. Some loss-making enterprises pay partial pensions and/or reimburse part of health expenditure (only medicine and/or expensive tests). Some loss-making units have nominal schemes but give no reimbursement.	Most units provide 50% reimbursement for health expenses for out- and in-patient services. Some loss-making enterprises pay partial pensions and/or reimburse part of health expenditure (just medicine and/or expensive tests). Some loss-making units have nominal scheme but give no reimbursement
Others		
Beneficiaries	Commercial insurance, student insurance and rural Cooperative Medical System. Principally peasants and students. Commercial insurance has no special target population.	As for Nantong. As for Nantong.
Source of finance	Mainly from participants. CMS may receive some support from collectives.	As for Nantong.
Benefits	Commercial insurance pays reimbursement according to the premium and insurance contract. The focus is typically on large expenditure or specified items. CMS reimburses both out-patient and in-patient services, but usually at low rates.	As for Nantong.

Table 4.15 presents data on the kinds of employee in the sample institutions. Employees of government and public agency employees tend to have permanent posts. Enterprises in the category 'other', on the other hand, largely employ people on fixed-term contracts or temporary workers.

Table 4.15 Composition of employees by employment type, Nantong

Type of unit	Employment type			
	Permanent	Contracted	Temporary	Retiree
Government and public agencies	64.2	0.9	0.3	34.6
SOEs	28.0	45.2	0.7	26.1
COEs	15.9	58.1	0.6	24.8
Other ownership enterprises	8.7	70.2	15.5	5.6

Government and public agencies have the highest proportion of retirees, followed by SOEs and COEs. The former units reported that 36.2 per cent of their workforce (including retirees) were over 60 years of age (Table 4.16). SOEs also reported substantial numbers in this category. The other kinds of enterprise had a much younger workforce. This difference reflects the history of different categories of enterprise. Many government and public agencies and SOEs were established years ago and their workforce has aged. Most of the other enterprises were established since 1990. This is one reason why their workforce is younger. Another reason is that they have few permanent staff.

Table 4.16 Composition of employees by age, Nantong

Type of institution	Age			
	<40	40–60	60–80	>80
Government and public agencies	28.8	35.1	32.4	3.8
SOEs	32.8	37.0	25.1	1.5
COEs	48.3	32.4	18.5	0.8
Other ownership enterprises	85.2	11.0	3.6	0.2

Table 4.17 Unit-paid medical fees as percentage of total salary, Nantong

Type of institutions	Expenditure on medical benefits as a percentage of total salary	
	1995	1996
Government and public agencies	16.3	16.9
SOEs	11.4	10.5
COEs	10.1	12.0
Other ownership	3.6	4.0

Table 4.17 presents data on the cost of health benefits as a percentage of total salary in the years just before the launch of the municipal health insurance scheme.

Government and public agencies spent 16.9 per cent of salaries, SOEs and COEs spent a lower proportion and other enterprises spent very little on health. The differences reflect the age profile and benefits packages of the categories of employer. LIS schemes tend to demand smaller co-payments for those with long years of service (Table 4.18). This is another reason why enterprises with an older workforce tend to spend more on health benefits.

Table 4.18 Rates of co-payment by enterprise-based LIS, Nantong

Enterprise	Rate of co-payment for those with different length of service (%)				
	<10 years	10–20 years	20–30 years	>30 years	Retired
Unit A	25	20	15	10	5
Unit B	20	15	10	10	8
Unit C	25	20	15	10	10
Unit D	22	20	18	16	16

Nantong Municipal Health Insurance Scheme

Nantong launched its municipal health insurance scheme in 1997. All government and public agencies, and enterprises were invited to join. Employers contributed a premium (11.5 per cent of previous year's salary when the scheme was introduced in 1997, reduced to 8 per cent in 2000) and individuals contributed to their individual account (1 per cent of the previous year's salary in 1997, increased to 2 per cent in 2000).

Initially, individuals were expected to fund minor illnesses out of their individual account, supplemented by out-of-pocket payments. After spending 5 per cent of the previous year's salary people could claim reimbursement from the social risk fund, with some co-payment. A small number of people with special entitlements (war veterans, retired cadres and so forth) could claim reimbursement for all medical expenses. The government established a Health Insurance Fund Administration to manage the scheme.

By the end of 1998 the scheme was experiencing serious financial difficulties. The individual accounts had a notional balance of CNY24 million, but the social risk fund had a deficit of CNY43 million, of which CNY15 million had been used to finance health care for people with special entitlements. The net deficit was CNY17 million.

Table 4.19 Age composition of employees and type of health care, Nantong

Type of health care	Age (%)			
	<40	40–60	60–80	>80
Municipal health insurance	36.6	31.3	30.8	3.3
LIS	50.3	38.3	11.4	0.2
Commercial insurance	99.3	0.7	0.0	0.0

The study took place in late 1999. At that time, eight units were in the scheme, 12 had remained in LIS and one had joined a commercial insurance scheme. The enterprises that joined the municipal scheme tended to have an older workforce (Table 4.19). It is particularly notable that a much higher proportion of their workforce (working and retired) were over 60 years of age and 3.3 per cent were over 80. Enterprises that did not join had a younger workforce. Enterprises that joined the scheme tended to have a much higher proportion of permanent staff and many more retirees (Table 4.20).

Table 4.20 Type of employment and type of health care, Nantong

Type of health care	Employment type (%)			
	Permanent	Contracted	Temporary	Retiree
Municipal health insurance	47.5	12.0	6.7	33.8
LIS	18.6	66.9	1.9	18.6
Commercial insurance	0.0	100.0	0.0	0.0

Table 4.21 presents data on expenditure on the health benefit as a percentage of total salary. Institutions that joined the scheme reported high levels of health expenditure before joining (16.5 per cent) and a subsequent fall. Institutions that did not join reported lower levels of expenditure on health benefits before and after the municipal scheme was launched.

Table 4.21 Expenditure on health benefits as percentage of total salary, Nantong

Form of insurance	Expenditure on health benefits as percentage of total salary			
	1995	1996	1997	1998
Municipal health insurance	16.5*	16.5*	12.3	13.2
LIS	9.1	9.1	9.3	8.9
Commercial insurance	1.6	1.6	1.1	1.0

*Before joining the scheme.

Table 4.22 Types of employment in SOEs joining/not joining the municipal insurance scheme, Nantong

Type of SOE	Municipal scheme	Type of employment (%)			
		Permanent	Contracted	Temporary	Retiree
Profit-making	Joined	62.5	36.2	4.7	32.7
	Not joined	42.5	45.7	0.3	11.5
Loss-making	Joined	33.3	34.1	0.2	32.5
	Not joined	0.0	72.2	0.2	27.6

Tables 4.22 and 4.23 look particularly at the SOEs, distinguishing between profit-making and loss-making enterprises. The enterprises that joined had a higher percentage of permanent employees and retirees, a higher portion of elder employees and higher spending on medical care. It is particularly noteworthy that the loss-making enterprises that joined the scheme had been spending a very high proportion of salary costs on health benefits.

Table 4.23 Age of workforce and cost of medical benefit in SOEs joining/not joining the municipal insurance scheme, Nantong

Type of SOE	Municipal scheme	Age of workforce (%)				Medical benefit as % of salary	
		<40	40–60	60–80	>80	1995	1996
Profit-making	Joined	39.0	37.2	19.3	4.5	9.2	9.6
	Not joined	45.0	45.3	9.7	0.0	7.8	7.3
Loss-making	Joined	36.3	34.6	27.3	1.8	20.5	19.2
	Not joined	35.6	48.4	15.7	0.3	11.5	8.8

Focus group discussions with enterprise managers and employees revealed that they assessed potential benefits and costs when deciding whether to join the municipal health insurance scheme. Box 4.1 summarizes the discussions at one enterprise (E) that joined the scheme and one (F) that did not. Both discussions revealed serious doubts about the usefulness of the scheme. Many of these issues were addressed when the scheme was redesigned in mid-2000.

Box 4.1 Attitudes to the municipal insurance scheme in Nantong, late 1999

Unit E

This was a loss-making enterprise. After joining the scheme, the enterprise had to spend more on medical care than previously. In 1995 and 1996, the enterprise sent 11.5 per cent and 11.6 per cent of total salary; in 1997 and 1998, after joining the scheme, it spent 11.9 per cent and 12.2 per cent of total salary. The employees had to pay more out of pocket according to the regulations of the scheme. They were less likely to visit hospitals than before, preferring to buy drugs from pharmacies for minor illnesses. Since joining the scheme, the number of health professionals working at the enterprise clinic fell from four to two, owing largely to a fall in utilization.

Unit F

This was a profitable enterprise with a relatively young workforce. Between 1995 and 1998, its annual spending on health care was 8.4 per cent, 5.6 per cent, 4.9 per cent and 7.7 per cent of total salary. The enterprise did not join the scheme because it would have had to pay more in contributions, whilst the benefits to employees would diminish, and the employees would have to choose from a limited list of health providers.

Nantong modified the design of the scheme in July 2000. The main changes were:

- The employer's contribution was decreased from 11.8 per cent to 8 per cent of average salary;
- The individual's contribution was increased from 1 to 2 per cent of salary;
- The employer's contribution for retirees was set at 2 per cent of pension to be paid into individual accounts;
- Funding from the social risk fund was only to be used for in-patient care and certain chronic conditions. Individuals would use their savings accounts for out-patient care;
- Special funds were available for catastrophic illness (when expenditure exceeded CNY30,000 in a year);
- Employers were permitted to purchase supplementary insurance;
- The entitlements for the special group were to be paid from a government grant equivalent to CNY4,100 per person.

A report by the Nantong Health Insurance Management Centre (2001) suggests that these changes were successful. More loss-making enterprises could afford to join the scheme. The provision for catastrophic illness protected against serious impoverishment. After the modification the scheme increased the number of beneficiaries and improved its financial situation. Between April 1997 and June 2000, 853 units with 71,000 employees had joined the scheme; total income was CNY228.14 million and total spending was CNY219.65 million. By June 2001, 1,890 units with 255,000 employees were members of the scheme; total income for the year following July 2000 was CNY116.88 million and total spending was CNY76.69 million. It remains to be seen if the new arrangements are sustainable and if they provide adequate coverage for beneficiaries.

Health Sector Reform

This section outlines the major health system reforms that have taken place in the two cities.

Nantong

Discussions with local health officials, hospital managers and informants in the Nantong Health Insurance Management Centre revealed the following problems in Nantong:

- *Insufficient government health investment.* This obliges hospitals to depend chiefly on their health service income. Hospitals make all sorts of provisions to finance the purchase of sophisticated equipment as a source of revenue. This has contributed to cost increases.
- *Health pricing system.* Prices are still set by government. Many health services are priced lower than their cost, but new technologies have quite high prices.

This has led facilities to rely on drug sales and sophisticated clinical tests as sources of revenue.
- *Inappropriate mix of facilities.* Downtown Nantong is well supplied with referral hospitals, but has few primary health care facilities. Most medical services are provided by referral hospitals.
- *Problems of the poor and vulnerable.* Certain social groups are experiencing difficulty in accessing medical care. These include unemployed and laid-off workers and rural-to-urban migrants.

In recent years, the Nantong government has undertaken a series of health reforms focusing on personnel administration; hospital management; municipal health insurance, community health services and disease prevention.

Reforming personnel administration
Graduates of medical colleagues in Nantong were previously assigned to health facilities. They now must sit an examination to test whether they are qualified for the post. Employees were previously assigned a job title based on their qualifications and position. Now people have to compete for promotion posts. This encourages all health workers to work harder. An employee who breaks a health regulation may be dismissed from his or her current position and will have to await another opportunity.

Hospital management
By the end of 2001, Nantong had categorized all its hospitals as either profit-making or not-for-profit. It had established pricing, taxation and other policies to govern the different types of hospital. Some new private hospitals opened in the development zone of Nantong. The government introduced procedures to reduce the incentives for hospitals to sell drugs by requiring not-for-profit hospitals to transfer all revenues from drug sales to a specific bank account controlled by the Municipal Finance Bureau. They, in turn, were allocated a share of the pooled revenue. The government also introduced multi-institutional competitive tendering for drugs.

Improvement of the urban health insurance reform
Nantong launched a city-wide employment-based health insurance scheme (HIS) in early 1997. By the end of 1999 only 20 per cent of employees were covered. In early 2000 the policy was adjusted by reducing the contributions from 12.5 per cent of salary to 10 per cent and by extending coverage to laid-off and unemployed workers, with no contribution. By the end of 2002 the scheme covered 95 per cent of employees in downtown Nantong.

Regional health plan
In early 2001 the municipal government requested the health department to develop a regional health plan to rationalize health services. The plan was finished and approved by government later that year. It now provides the framework for allocating health resources in the city.

Community health service system

The community health services were the weakest part of the health system in downtown Nantong. The regional health plan drew attention to the need to strengthen the community health system. In late 2002 the Health Bureau and the Bureau of Labour and Social Security jointly issued a document encouraging HIS participants to attend community health centres by offering an additional reimbursement of 5 per cent for people who used this level of care.

Separation of disease prevention and surveillance

Previously, disease control and prevention and the enforcement of public health laws were integrated in preventive facilities, such as AESs and health bureaux. These two functions have been separated and fall under the remit of two institutions, the CDC and the Institute of Health Surveillance.

Further reforms

The Nantong government is planning to implement further reforms in two major fields:

- *Reorganization of medical resources.* The municipal government has recently issued a formal document to launch the regional health plan. This work has been assigned to the municipal Health Bureau. The Health Bureau is proposing a reorganization of health resources in downtown Nantong. The key points of the proposal are to adjust the service functions of each health facility and merge some hospitals to form medical groups. The Municipal Health Bureau has been trying to establish a unified system for hospital logistical services to reduce costs and improve resource allocation.
- *Privatizing public health facilities.* Almost all the township health centres in six counties had changed their ownership by the end of 2002. The government constructed an independent preventive health facility in each township to undertake preventive and MCH services and rural health surveillance. This process has not begun in downtown Nantong.

Zibo

According to key informant interviews with officials from the Health, Labour and Social Security, and Civil Affairs Bureaux as well as with hospital managers, enterprise managers and community representatives, the major health sector problems are as follows:

- *Cost escalation of medical services.* Cost escalation has become the most serious problem in health care in Zibo. Causes of cost escalation in Zibo were largely attributed to the inflation of medical supplies and to the use of sophisticated equipment and expensive drugs. Drug expenses accounted for at least 50 per cent of total medical expenditures and the use of high-tech diagnostic and treatment services is very common.

- *Inefficient health service provision.* Inefficient service provision is widespread. Key people from the municipal Bureau of Health emphasized that average hospital out-patient visits and hospital bed-days were not increased in line with the number of hospital personnel and other resources. This was attributed to the imbalance between demand for health care and the development of health care services.
- *Access to health care.* The income gap between the poor and the rich has widened in recent years in Zibo. Besides significant differences between rural and urban populations in income and other indicators of economic and social status, within the urban environment the gaps between different population groups have also increased. In Zibo the 'vulnerable' urban population (the laid-off and unemployed, the elderly, the disabled, indigents and the floating population) are experiencing difficulty in accessing basic health services because they simply cannot afford them.
- *Pricing policy.* After the changes in pricing policy in 1980 from a low-price policy to a cost-based pricing policy, user charges have been the major source of finance for public hospitals. Prices are fixed by the provincial government, which constrains the autonomy of the municipal government in setting and regulating its own prices.
- *Payment systems.* Fee-for-service is still the main payment method in the urban health insurance scheme. Problems of cost escalation and the provision of unnecessary care are closely related to this payment system. The Zibo government has not radically changed the urban health insurance schemes; hence the introduction of new payment methods has been thwarted.

In order to address the above problems, a number of health sector reforms have been taken in Zibo. These reforms include:

Hospital reimbursement system reform
From 1980, in line with China's economic reform, the local government in Zibo began to reform the reimbursement methods for hospitals. The major features of the reform are: substantial increases of user fees; hospitals can retain all the surplus of revenues generated for their own development; and, in general, hospitals now have more economic autonomy. As a result, user charges have become a major source of hospital revenue.

Government urban health insurance reform
In order to control the escalation of medical costs and sustain the existing government urban health insurance scheme, Zibo's government initiated health insurance reform in 1994. 1,608 institutions and 105,000 employees are involved in this scheme. This reform has modified the traditional insurance financing mechanism. In central cities, 11 per cent of total salaries are collected as the insurance fund, about 20 per cent of which come from individual employees. In county cities, 10 per cent of salaries are collected. A health insurance fund management organization has been established in each district and county. Hospitals which meet certain set price levels and standards of service quality are

eligible for contracts from the insurance management organization. If the contract hospitals provide treatment over and above these agreed services, the fund administrative agent will refuse to pay the costs. The reform also established a referral system.

Regional health resource planning
In 1992 the Zhoucun district of Zibo was involved in an experiment to reform the existing pattern of health resource allocation, in an effort to increase efficiency and equity. The reform package granted local government the authority to plan the distribution of available health resources regardless of the ownership of the resources. By doing this, it was hoped that the duplication of facilities and functions would be avoided and more resources could be transferred from high-level hospitals to community health centres. However, to date this reform has not achieved its expected outcome owing to the political and administrative complexities of the health resource management system.

Community health care system reform
Since 1980, the community health care system in urban cities has been largely destroyed owing primarily to an increase in hospital autonomy and the cancellation of the referral system. An inadequate community health care system is one reason for the rapid increase in medical costs, and its re-establishment is one of the strategies being employed to combat unreasonable medical fee escalation. Community health centres and stations have been established which provide curative and preventive services. These centres are successfully recruiting newly trained health workers from hospitals. The success of this reform will benefit both regional health resource planning and health insurance reform, because the redistribution of health resources will increase the efficiency of the health system. However, it is understood that developing the community health sector will take a long time and it is expected that political support for the initiative should be cumulative.

Further reforms
At the time of this report, two main health sector reforms are planned by the Zibo government. One is to reform the ownership system of the public hospitals. The second is to continue to reform the urban health insurance scheme:

* *Hospital sector ownership system reform*. Undertaken by Zibo's municipal government in accordance with guidelines from central and provincial government. Hospitals within Zibo will be divided up, according to their particular functions and sources of finance, into two categories: not-for-profit hospitals and for-profit hospitals. Different financial and pricing policies will be implemented in each type of hospital, and service provision and target population will be clearly defined.
* *Implementation of the urban health insurance scheme*. Reform was to commence on 1 January 1999, according to the agenda laid down by the state government. In Shandong Province, five cities were to have begun

implementing reforms on this date; other cities, including Zibo, were to do so six months later on 1 July 1999. However, for various reasons, the implementation of urban health insurance reform in Zibo was delayed until early 2002. The following changes have been made to the benefit package: unemployed workers are offered special government subsidies for their insurance and hence will be able to obtain a basic health insurance package. One disadvantageous change is that patients suffering catastrophic diseases will bear heavy economic burdens because a ceiling will be set in the new health insurance scheme. A specific administrative unit is to be established within the Bureau of Labour and Social Security.

Table 4.24 summarizes the health sector reforms that the Zibo and Nantong municipal governments are implementing.

Table 4.24 Summary of health sector reforms in Zibo and Nantong

Type of reform	Key aspects	Comments
Personnel administration	Recruitment Promotion	Moving away from permanent employment.
Hospital management	Reduce government share in total hospital revenues. Increase financial autonomy of hospitals. Adjust prices of medical services. De-link hospital revenue from drug sales.	Hospitals depend much more on the market.
Urban health insurance reform	Pool the urban health insurance fund across the municipal city. Collect funds from both employees and employers. Change payment methods. Set co-payment.	Cost contained. Affect utilization of health service by the poor.
Regional health planning	Improve resource allocation. Control equipment of high technologies. Reduce duplication of health facilities and services.	Cost contained.
Community health care system	Reallocate health resources from high level health facilities to primary health care units. Expand network of primary care facilities. Control costs through establishing referral system.	Improve access to health services and control costs.
Separation of disease prevention and surveillance	Improve preventive health services. Strengthen enforcement of laws.	Strengthen prevention.

Chapter 5

Access to and Use of Health Care Services by Employees and Their Families

Henry Lucas, Jiaying Chen and Zhonghua Weng

The economic reform process in China, which started in the early 1980s, has resulted in an extended period of rapid growth that has substantially increased the incomes of a majority of the population. But for a sizeable minority the benefits have been much more limited. Both inter-regional and inter-household income inequalities have increased sharply and there are many people still living in poverty (see, for example, *China Rural Statistics Yearbook*, 1999). These inequalities are reflected in dramatic differences in the health status of those living in poor and rich areas (Hao *et al.*, 1994). One important contributory factor has been a pronounced rise in the cost of access to health services.

In line with the general transition towards a more market-oriented economy, health facilities have become increasingly dependent on user charges. With a declining share of their revenue being derived from government subsidies, facility managers have now acquired considerable autonomy, and health authorities have difficulty in exercising effective regulatory control. This has contributed to rapid cost increases, as facilities have responded to incentives to increase their revenue from drug sales and diagnostic tests (Chen *et al.*, 1999).

In urban areas, the nature of service provision varies widely between different localities. In some cities, traditional enterprise-based facilities remain an important source of care. In others, there has been a rapid growth in private clinics and drug stores. However, partly due to the perceived poor quality of services at primary level (Hao *et al.*, 1999), the general tendency has been towards an escalating use of municipal hospital services, even for routine out-patient care. This has again exacerbated the upward pressure on costs. One government response has been to pilot supply-side reforms, including the development of new models of community-based care designed to draw patients away from hospital out-patient departments. However, these initiatives have been limited in scope and their eventual impact remains uncertain.

The health care expenditures of many urban employees and retired workers are subsidized by benefits derived from their work unit. Until recently, the schemes providing such benefits could mainly be classified under two broad headings. The government insurance system (GIS) was for government employees, and the labour insurance system (LIS) provided for workers in state-owned enterprises. The GIS was funded out of government budgets and LIS out of enterprise welfare funds. However, since the mid-1990s a number of cities (including those discussed in this book) have launched municipal employment-based health insurance schemes (HIS), which all government agencies, public institutions and enterprises were invited to join. (National Committee of Administrative System Reform of China, 1996). The various schemes are outlined in Chapter 4 but it should be noted that, as with other aspects of social provision in China, the details may vary substantially between locations and, in the case of LIS, between individual enterprises.

Rising health costs have considerably increased the financial burden both on enterprises and government (Meng *et al.*, 2002) and on households and individuals. Large and growing numbers of people work for loss-making enterprises which are finding it increasingly difficult to meet the cost of health care benefits. Others work for small companies which do not provide health insurance. In many cities there is also a growing population of unofficial rural-to-urban migrant residents (usually described as the floating population) who have no entitlement to health care. The National Health Services Survey (NHSS) indicates that the proportion of people in urban areas covered by insurance decreased substantially from 72 per cent to 56 per cent between 1993 and 1998 (Gao *et al.*, 2001) and that those not covered are experiencing great difficulty in gaining access to care.

It is recognized that increasing inequalities in access to services could not only have serious consequences for health but may also reduce public support for the economic reform process. Given that serious problems exist for a substantial and increasing proportion of those living in urban areas, the effective targeting of government initiatives designed to improve this situation has become a core policy issue (Oxaal and Cook, 1998). The main aim of this and the following chapter will be to explore issues associated with targeting in relation to health care provision, focusing on the identification of those in greatest need. Here, the focus will be on those in formal employment and their households. In Chapter 6, other sections of the population will be considered.

Background to the Study

A study was carried out over the period 1998–2001 to consider the implications of the introduction of new forms of health financing scheme and explore the relationship between transition, health reform and health system performance in urban areas. The research was developed in consultation with the Ministry of Health, which had identified a need for systematic evidence on how changes in health finance had affected the performance of urban health services in both equity and efficiency. In collaboration with the Ministry, two in-depth case studies of medium-sized cities were designed and implemented, one in Nantong in Jiangsu Province and the other in Zibo in Shandong Province. The cities were seen as similar to many others in the eastern provinces of China in population size and economic status. They were also regarded as of particular interest because their governments had actively supported innovative approaches to health system development.

Progress in the two cities over the reform period has varied considerably. Nantong has experienced relatively rapid economic development based largely on the emergence of new enterprises, including a number involving joint ventures with international companies. The booming economy has proved very attractive to migrant labour, and there is a registered floating population of over 250,000. Zibo, on the other hand, has been hampered by the financial difficulties experienced by the large number of long-established SOEs. Around 20 per cent were effectively bankrupt in 1999 and 450,000 people were registered as unemployed. A considerable proportion of the population live in agricultural households and find it very difficult to obtain formal employment in government or state enterprises.

Partly in consequence of its relative prosperity, Nantong has a well-developed municipal health insurance system that covered around 95 per cent of employees in 2002. Those within this scheme are generally seen as having good access to care, much of which is provided by higher level municipal hospitals. Most enterprise clinics are small and provide only basic services. The level of coverage and source of provision has driven up treatment costs, such that many of those excluded from the HIS or similar schemes either have problems gaining access or are forced to spend a high proportion of their income on health care. In Zibo, by contrast, though an HIS was launched in 1999, only a small minority of the population are covered, and these are mainly employees in government agencies and public institutions. Overall, a much smaller proportion of the population has good health care coverage, greater use is made of enterprise and private clinics, and the average cost of care is much lower.

This chapter considers the experience of those people in Nantong and Zibo who are either formal sector employees or members of the household of such an employee. It attempts to assess the variation in their health care needs, demand for and access to services and the extent to which these are influenced by the type or effectiveness of the health care scheme to which that employee belongs.

Definition and Selection of Work Units and Employees

A cluster sample of employees was taken, based on lists of formal sector work units in each city. These were stratified under five broad headings: government agencies and public institutions; profitable SOEs; loss-making SOEs; COEs; and other enterprises. The definitions of these strata are:

- *Government agencies and public institutions.* These were covered by the GIS prior to the introduction of the health insurance reforms and both their funding sources and the health benefits their employees enjoyed differed significantly from those associated with SOEs. After the implementation of the reforms, benefits converged but sources of finance continued to differ.
- *Profitable and loss-making SOEs.* All workers in SOEs are in principle covered by an LIS. However, the health benefits offered vary greatly, depending on the

enterprise's financial situation. These were therefore divided into two sub-categories, profitable and loss-making.

- *COEs*. These belong to collective institutions, such as street administrative committees or public institutions with collective property. They are advised by government to implement the GIS, but many prefer to adopt a range of less generous alternatives.
- *Others*. Other enterprises include those which are joint-venture, joint-stock, foreign-investor and privately run. Such enterprises are generally profitable and have usually developed their own health benefit packages. Some are implementing a version of LIS and offer similar benefits to those provided by the SOEs. However, others provide very limited cover or none at all.

Sample Design

The original sample design required a total of 20 enterprises to be selected: two government agencies/public institutions, four profitable SOEs, six loss-making SOEs, four collective enterprises and four others. Fifty employees were then to be randomly sampled from each work unit, leading to a total sample of 1,000 households. The criteria for selecting work units were as follows:

- Of the two government agencies and public institutions, one was to be a government agency, such as a municipal health bureau, and the other a public institution, such as a school or hospital. This was on the basis that the latter typically have more rigid constraints on the funding available for health care schemes. In Nantong it was difficult to find a government agency with 50 employees and therefore two agencies were sampled.
- Four profitable SOEs were to be selected from the most profitable in the city, two of these covered by the new health insurance scheme. It was assumed that these enterprises would have no financial constraints on the provision of generous health care cover.
- The six loss-making SOEs were to be operating at a loss but operating normally. At least three were to be participants in the new health insurance scheme, if applicable.
- Of the four collective enterprises selected, half should be participants in the new health insurance scheme. It was also thought desirable to include profitable, non-profitable and loss-making COEs in the sample.
- Of the four other enterprises included, one was joint-ventured, one joint-stock, one foreign-invested and one privately owned. If possible, one or two of the enterprises should be covered by the new scheme.

Approach to the Analysis

The survey can be seen as generating two distinct though closely related samples – one consisting of the employees themselves and the other of the members of their households, some employed in other work units. For employees, the exact nature of their work unit and health care scheme were known. For the larger sample it was necessary to rely on reported information on employment and cover. Where the sample size allows, the analysis examines both these groups.

One rationale for considering the various categories of work unit was an assumption that the nature of the benefits offered by the various health care schemes, HIS, GIS, LIS, etc., could vary considerably between one work unit and another. Knowing that an employee was in principle covered by the LIS provided by a given enterprise was not sufficient to understand the benefits available in practice. Most obviously, a loss-making enterprise might provide far worse cover than one which was profitable. In the analysis, therefore, it has proved useful to look at schemes from three different perspectives: the type of scheme, the type of work unit and, perhaps most importantly, the perceived quality of the benefits provided. This latter characterization was based on the perceptions of the selected employees in the case of the specific work units sampled, and the total household sample when considering all the work units in which they were employed. The classification involved a simple question as to whether the work unit scheme provided: appropriate assistance in a timely fashion; appropriate assistance but with considerably delay; no assistance or assistance which was substantially below entitlements.

Findings

Characteristics of Employees and Total Sample

Table 5.1 shows the age and sex distribution by type of work unit for the sampled employees in the two cities. Perhaps the most interesting characteristic of the table for Nantong is the high proportion (61 per cent) of women and those under 30 (41 per cent) in the 'Other' category – typically the newer, export-oriented joint enterprises. By comparison, only some 11–13 per cent of the SOE employees are under 30. Apart from the 'Other' category, women and men are more or less equally represented in each type of work unit. Note that less than 1 per cent of employees are over 60. As in Nantong, the main feature in Zibo is the high proportion of those under 30 (49 per cent) in the 'Other' category. However, probably reflecting the nature of the specific enterprises, women are here greatly outnumbered by men (36 per cent compared to 64 per cent). The proportion of the younger age band in other categories is somewhat higher than in Nantong, at 15–21 per cent. Again, apart from the 'Other' category, women and men are more or less equally represented in each type of work unit and there are almost no employees over 60.

Table 5.2 shows the age and sex distribution of all members of the sampled households for each type of work unit employing their primary income earner. In both cities the sample appears more or less evenly distributed across types of work unit, apart from the somewhat greater proportion of members, especially female members, in the 15–29 year age band.

Table 5.1 Age and sex distribution by type of work unit – employees (%)

			Government agency	Profitable SOE	Loss-making SOE	COE	Other
Nantong	Males	15–29	4	7	6	9	16
		30–44	18	22	26	26	18
		45–59	22	20	22	12	4
		60+	0	0	1	0	0
	Females	15–29	14	6	5	7	25
		30–44	30	33	34	38	30
		45–59	12	12	7	6	6
		60+	0	1	0	0	0
Zibo	Males	15–29	8	7	8	8	32
		30–44	35	32	25	34	28
		45–59	12	9	14	15	4
		60+	0	0	0	1	0
	Females	15–29	7	14	11	9	17
		30–44	31	28	38	29	18
		45–59	8	10	4	4	2
		60+	0	0	0	0	0

Table 5.2 Age and sex distribution by type of work unit – all (%)

			Government agency	Profitable SOE	Loss-making SOE	COE	Other
Nantong	Males	0–14	7	10	10	10	7
		15–29	9	9	6	8	12
		30–44	17	17	18	19	15
		45–59	13	12	12	9	11
		60+	1	3	3	3	4
	Females	0–14	9	6	8	8	8
		15–29	11	10	9	9	15
		30–44	18	17	19	20	14
		45–59	10	11	11	9	11
		60+	2	4	4	6	4
Zibo	Males	0–14	9	10	11	9	10
		15–29	6	9	10	10	18
		30–44	22	21	22	20	17
		45–59	10	8	8	8	8
		60+	0	0	1	1	2
	Females	0–14	10	11	8	10	7
		15–29	11	11	11	11	17
		30–44	24	20	20	20	12
		45–59	7	8	8	8	7
		60+	0	2	1	3	2

As might be expected, there is a clear relationship between household income status and the type of work unit of the sampled employee. Table 5.3 indicates that in Nantong the households of employees in government agencies, profitable SOEs or other enterprises are much less likely to have incomes close to the poverty line (PL) than those of loss-making or COE employees. This pattern also holds in Zibo. Indeed, there is a more marked contrast, with considerably more than 40 per cent of households of employees in loss-making or collective enterprises having per capita incomes less than twice the poverty line. This clearly indicates the generally greater prosperity of Nantong.

Table 5.3 Household poverty status of employees by type of work unit (%)

Poverty status		Government agency	Profitable SOE	Loss-making SOE	COE	Others
Nantong	<PL	–	0.5	1.0	–	–
	1–2PL	4.0	13.2	25.9	35.9	8.0
	2–3PL	20.8	44.7	47.1	41.0	27.6
	>3PL	75.2	41.6	25.9	23.1	64.3
Zibo	<PL	1.0	0.5	2.5	12.1	3.2
	1–2PL	–	13.7	43.9	48.4	25.7
	2–3PL	36.3	38.1	40.8	30.2	30.5
	>3PL	62.7	47.7	12.9	9.3	40.6

There is also a clear relationship between household poverty status and the type of health care scheme to which members belong. In Table 5.4 around 50 per cent of those in the HIS in Nantong and 56 per cent in Zibo are in households with per capita incomes more than three time the poverty line. On the other hand, more than one third of those without coverage have income just above the poverty line. Note that in Zibo a similar proportion of those with an employee covered by the LIS fall into this income band.

Table 5.4 Household poverty status of all members by scheme (%)

		Self-payment	HIS	GIS	LIS	H-LIS	H-GIS
Nantong	<PL	0.9	0.2	–	0.5	0.6	–
	1–2PL	34.4	15.7	19.0	19.2	26.9	14.2
	2–3PL	37.4	35.2	38.1	43.6	47.5	47.2
	>3PL	27.3	48.9	42.9	36.6	25.0	38.7
Zibo	<PL	8.7	0.4	–	3.0	3.7	–
	1–2PL	37.3	5.0	7.4	32.3	46.5	–
	2–3PL	31.7	38.4	59.3	36.4	43.6	–
	>3PL	22.3	56.2	33.3	28.3	6.2	–

Table 5.5 illustrates the tendency of household members to have similar health care coverage. In Nantong, some 56 per cent of the members of households of government agency employees have HIS coverage, almost twice the proportion for those of an employee of an SOE or other enterprise and almost four times that of collective employee households. In Zibo, 67 per cent of the members of households of government agency employees have HIS coverage and 60 per cent of those of an employee of an SOE or other enterprise are covered by the LIS. In contrast to the position in Nantong, a substantial proportion (20–30 per cent) of family members have no coverage, irrespective of the employees type of work unit.

Table 5.5 Health scheme coverage of household members by employee work unit (%)

		Government agency	Profitable SOE	Loss-making SOE	COE	Others
Nantong	Self-payment	8.3	7.8	8.8	9.8	16.1
	HIS	56.4	27.1	30.4	15.3	29.4
	GIS	3.0	2.0	2.5	1.6	1.3
	LIS	13.2	42.3	39.0	50.7	36.3
	H-LIS	8.3	19.7	12.7	21.1	12.2
	H-GIS	10.6	1.0	6.1	1.3	0.6
	CMS	0.3	0.0	0.1	0.2	0.9
	Other	0.0	0.2	0.4	0.2	3.2
Zibo	Self-payment	23.6	22.5	17.0	23.5	33.7
	HIS	67.3	2.0	3.9	3.1	5.5
	GIS	1.5	1.8	i.^	0.3	0.4
	LIS	6.5	63.6	61.6	39.6	60.1
	H-LIS	0.7	9.6	16.4	5.1	0.2
	CMS	0.0	0.0	0.0	28.3	0.0
	Other	0.4	0.5	0.1	0.2	0.2

Reported Assessment of Health Care Schemes

As discussed above, the underlying assumption of the work unit study was that the quality of health care schemes would vary considerably. Table 5.6 shows the assessments of their work unit scheme by the sampled employees. Clearly in Nantong, government agencies and public institutions are perceived to be performing extremely well – none of their employees had any complaints. 'Other' enterprises perform almost as well, with just two employees alleging delayed payments, and profitable SOEs also score highly. Only one employee of the latter claimed that due reimbursement had not been paid and just 10 out of 175 complained of delays. The picture becomes much more varied for loss-making SOEs and COEs. Three of the former gain a perfect rating, while the other three are clearly seen as providing highly unsatisfactory benefits. In the worst case, 65 per cent of employees said that payments are no longer paid and two of the three are living up to the expectation of less than 10 per cent of their employees.

Similarly, three of the COEs are performing extremely well but 64 per cent of the employees of the fourth claimed that payments were not being made.

Unlike the situation in Nantong, one of the two selected government agencies and public institutions in Zibo is perceived by around one-third of its employees to be delaying reimbursements. 'Other' enterprises again perform well, with just two employees alleging delayed payments. Profitable SOEs again score highly. Only three employees claimed that due reimbursement had not been paid and just 5 out of 186 complained of delays. Four of the six loss-making SOEs are assessed as performing poorly. One scheme appears to be no longer meeting its obligations, while 80–90 per cent of employees in two others complained of delayed payments. Those in collective enterprises fare better, though one scheme here is assessed by 43 per cent of employees as failing. Similarly, while 'other' enterprises generally score very highly, all the employees of one scheme agreed that was no longer providing assistance with health care costs.

Table 5.6 Assessment of schemes – employees in each work unit (%)

	Work unit	Nantong			Zibo		
		Timely	Delays	Unpaid	Timely	Delays	Unpaid
Government	All	100	0	0	85	15	0
	1	100	0	0	72	28	0
	2	100	0	0	96	4	0
	3	100	0	0	–	–	–
Profitable	All	94	5	1	96	3	2
SOE	1	94	6	0	94	4	2
	2	95	5	0	100	0	0
	3	100	0	0	90	6	4
	4	87	11	2	100	0	0
Loss-making	All	59	27	14	44	33	23
SOE	1	100	0	0	14	86	0
	2	100	0	0	100	0	0
	3	100	0	0	55	9	36
	4	34	60	6	2	0	98
	5	9	26	65	2	93	5
	6	6	72	21	90	8	2
COE	All	75	8	17	90	1	9
	1	100	0	0	57	0	43
	2	98	2	0	97	3	0
	3	6	30	64	100	0	0
	4	100	0	0	96	2	2
Other	All	99	1	0	71	2	28
	1	100	0	0	95	5	0
	2	98	2	0	0	0	100
	3	100	0	0	100	0	0
	4	98	2	0	98	2	0

This pattern is confirmed by the recorded assessments of the total sample of employee household members as seen in Table 5.7. (Note that the description of their work unit here relies on the judgement of the respondent). In Nantong, loss-making SOEs are regarded as performing well by around 65 per cent of their employees while 13 per cent claim that they are not providing assistance. The corresponding figures for COEs is around 74 per cent and 15 per cent. As might be expected, given the greater number of work units covered, a small but substantial proportion, around 10 per cent of employees of profitable and 'other' enterprises have some complaint. However, government agencies and public institutions retain an almost perfect rating, with just seven complaints of delay and one of non-payment. In Zibo, problems are mainly confined to the unprofitable SOEs and 'other' enterprises.

Table 5.7 Assessment of insurance schemes – all (%)

	Nantong			Zibo		
	Timely	Delays	Unpaid	Timely	Delays	Unpaid
Government	97	3	0	84	15	1
Profitable SOE	87	8	5	93	4	3
Loss-making SOE	65	22	13	53	29	18
COE	74	11	15	87	2	11
Others	91	5	3	70	6	24

Heath Care Needs

Acute illness
Table 5.8 shows self-reported acute illness episodes by age and sex for both the employee and overall sample. In Nantong, the rates increase considerably with age, with those for the 45–59 year age bands being at least twice those of those aged 15–29. This trend continues with the overall sample, where rates for those over 60 are around 70 episodes per 100 persons in Nantong. Interestingly, reported illness rates are generally substantially higher for women in all age bands except for those under 15. In Zibo, rates for those over 60 are less than in Nantong, at around 55 episodes per 100 persons. Reported illness rates for women are again higher except for those under 15 or over 60. Note that rates for employees are considerably higher than those for all household members. This probably reflects the central role taken by the employee in the study, though it is not clear if this has resulted in an over-reporting of their own sickness or an under-reporting of the illness episodes of other household members.

Table 5.8 Acute illness episodes in two-week reference period by age (/100 persons)

		Employees			Total sample		
		Male	Female	All	Male	Female	All
Nantong	0–14	–	–	–	43	35	39
	15–29	30	47	39	21	35	29
	30–44	47	60	55	36	49	42
	45–59	79	96	85	60	64	62
	60+	–	–	–	72	63	67
	All	55	63	59	42	48	45
Zibo	0–14	–	–	–	27	27	27
	15–29	27	19	23	18	13	16
	30–44	31	44	37	26	36	30
	45–59	34	42	37	28	33	30
	60+	–	–	–	55	56	56
	All	31	38	34	25	29	27

Chronic illness
Table 5.9 considers expenditure on the treatment of chronic conditions by employees and all household members. In Nantong, the overall median expenditure and reimbursement rate are both higher for employees in government agencies and profitable SOEs than for those in unprofitable enterprises. However, the differences are limited. For the overall sample, there is little variation across the range of work unit categories.

Table 5.9 Expenditure over previous year on chronic illness by work unit

	Nantong			Zibo		
	Median spent	Median repaid (%)	Cases	Median spent	Median repaid (%)	Cases
Employees						
Government agency	340	75	16	1,500	80	14
Profitable SOE	450	85	67	600	50	35
Loss-making SOE	300	67	62	500	0	45
COE	325	70	44	600	0	25
Other	270	90	31	700	0	9
All	390	80	220	625	0	128
Total sample						
Government agency	500	75	46	1,200	50	25
Profitable SOE	500	80	179	500	0	79
Loss-making SOE	500'	55	172	600	0	106
COE	500	36	134	675	0	56
Other	450	83	101	700	0	33
All	500	70	632	600	0	299

The median expenditure for profitable enterprises is reported to be the same as that for loss-making enterprises even though the reimbursement rate for the latter is much lower. Overall it would seem that employees and their households generally meet the cost of care for chronic illness even if the support they receive is limited. The situation appears similar in Zibo. Again, there are considerable variations in reimbursement rates between different work units but this appears to have little impact on overall expenditures. Reimbursement rates are markedly lower than in Nantong, apart from those for government agencies. Expenditures for the latter appear substantially higher, though the low numbers limit the significance of this finding.

Hospitalization

While the cost of treatment for acute and even chronic illness may be relatively manageable for those in households where at least one member is formally employed, the costs of hospitalization are typically of a different order of magnitude. The tables in this section examine the proportion of those referred by a doctor who enter hospital. Note that given that the number of employees referred to hospital was very low, only the overall sample is considered. In Table 5.10, the first observation is that the number of referrals in Nantong is considerably higher than in Zibo. This is particularly evident for profitable SOEs, but similar referral rates hold for COEs and 'other' enterprises, though not for government agencies. This may indicate a greater willingness to propose hospitalization where coverage and general incomes make it more affordable. This high referral rate may explain the otherwise surprising finding that the proportion of those referred entering hospital in Nantong is considerably lower for those in households with an employee in a profitable SOE. In Zibo, the proportion entering hospital is higher for those in households with an employee in a profitable SOE or 'other' enterprises. However, with the small number of hospitalizations, interpretation is problematic.

Table 5.10 Entered hospital when referred (%) by work unit – total sample

	Nantong			Zibo		
	Number of referrals	Referrals (% sample)	Entered hospital (%)	Number of referrals	Referrals (% sample)	Entered hospital (%)
Government agency	10	3.30	50	10	3.56	50
Profitable SOE	48	7.78	50	19	3.35	84
Loss-making SOE	44	4.76	73	35	3.77	63
COE	43	6.77	44	22	3.32	50
Other	46	6.71	78	21	3.98	90
All	191	6.03	61	107	3.61	68

Health Service Utilization

Acute illness

Table 5.11 would suggest that the type of work unit has little impact on the decision to seek health care for an acute illness. Though government agencies are seen as providing good health care schemes in Nantong, both the employee and overall samples for this category make the lowest use of health care services. Otherwise the rates vary little, though the proportions for loss-making SOEs are also somewhat lower than for other categories. In Zibo, the table does appear to indicate that both employees and household members have higher utilization rates for profitable SOEs. However, though government agencies are also generally perceived as providing good health care schemes, both the employee and overall samples for this category make the lowest use of health care services. In general, the rates do not vary dramatically.

Table 5.11 Visited doctor when sick in two-week reference period by work unit (%)

		Nantong	Zibo
Employees	Government agency	31	39
	Profitable SOE	45	64
	Loss-making SOE	39	49
	COE	51	54
	Others	73	42
	All	48	52
Total sample	Government agency	27	42
	Profitable SOE	46	58
	Loss-making SOE	36	50
	COE	45	55
	Others	48	48
	All	42	52

Table 5.12 Visited doctor when sick in two-week reference period by scheme (%)

		Nantong	Zibo
Employees	GIS and HIS	45	39
	LIS	50	52
	Other	83	88
	All	48	53
Total sample	GIS and HIS	41	45
	LIS	43	49
	Other	47	66
	Self-payment	24	57
	All	42	52

Again, though those who have to meet their own health care costs are much less likely to seek care in Nantong, the type of scheme to which they belong seems to have very limited impact (Table 5.12). The position is similar in Zibo. However, in this case the utilization rate is much the same even where payment for services is out of pocket.

Table 5.13 compares those in satisfactory (timely reimbursement) schemes to all others. In Nantong, there does appear to be some limited effect of belonging to a failing health care scheme. The latter seem to have utilization rates which are some 20–40 per cent lower. In Zibo, on the other hand, there seems little effect and no consistent pattern for either sample.

Table 5.13 Visited doctor when sick in two-week reference period by coverage (%)

			0–14	15–29	30–44	45–59	60+	All
Employees	Nantong	Timely	–	53	50	49	–	50
		Other	–	43	29	49	–	41
	Zibo	Timely	–	59	56	31	–	53
		Other	–	27	49	50	–	47
Total	Nantong	Timely	42	56	46	46	36	46
sample		Other	50	29	28	34	22	32
	Zibo	Timely	61	55	55	33	35	51
		Other	67	38	46	50	40	48

Table 5.14 Expenditure over previous year on chronic illness by scheme

		Nantong			Zibo		
		Median spent	Median repaid (%)	Cases	Median spent	Median repaid (%)	Cases
Employees	GIS and HIS	300	87	116	1,000	80	18
	LIS	500	70	100	600	0	109
	All	390	80	220	63	0	127
Total	GIS and HIS	400	85	229	1,000	75	36
sample	LIS	500	70	319	600	0	210
	Other	600	53	38	600	0	6
	Self-payment	375	0	46	1,000	0	47
	All	500	70	632	600	0	299

Though reimbursement rates in Nantong are seen to vary considerably by scheme (Table 5.14), this seems in general to have very little relationship to health care expenditures. The findings in Zibo seem to confirm the high reimbursements and expenditures associated with the GIS and HIS schemes. For both samples, only a minority with LIS coverage received any reimbursement and this is reflected in the total expenditure. Again, those paying out of pocket tend to contradict this finding, reporting a similar expenditure. However, the number is small and it is possible that this group may be especially prone to overstatement.

Table 5.15 considers the same issue, but focuses on the quality of the health care scheme provided. Again, even where no reimbursement is forthcoming the median expenditure on care appears to be maintained.

Table 5.15 Expenditure over previous year on chronic illness by coverage

		Nantong			Zibo		
		Median spent	Median repaid (%)	Cases	Median spent	Median repaid (%)	Cases
Employees	Timely	300	85	169	600	0	94
	Other	484	0	51	700	0	33
	All	390	80	220	600	0	127
Total	Timely	500	80	438	600	0	178
sample	Other	500	0	146	800	0	74
	All	500	75	584	600	0	252

Table 5.16, on the other hand, would appear to support the hypothesis that membership of the 'improved' HIS (or GIS – as indicated above, the GIS and HIS provide similar benefits) in Nantong does encourage a greater willingness to accept a referral to hospital. Around 75 per cent of those covered by the HIS or GIS enter hospital compared with 50 per cent of those covered by an LIS. (Note that, contrary to expectations, a similar proportion of those paying the full cost of care enter hospital, though the numbers are very small.) In Zibo, membership of the new scheme does not necessarily increase the admittance rate, though the numbers are small. Around 65 per cent of those covered by the LIS enter hospital compared with 50 per cent of those covered by the GIS/HIS. As in Nantong, the admittance rate for those paying the full cost of hospital care is high.

Table 5.16 Entered hospital when referred (%) by scheme – total sample

	Nantong		Zibo	
	Entered hospital (%)	Number of referrals	Entered hospital (%)	Number of referrals
GIS and HIS	73	77	50	10
LIS	50	82	65	65
Other	50	18	100	1
Self-payment	71	14	78	27
All	61	191	68	68

Finally, Table 5.17 provides limited supporting evidence that belonging to a failing scheme in Nantong tends to discourage the use of health care services, with the proportion of those in such schemes apparently much less likely to enter hospital. Once again there seems to be no indication that this has any effect in Zibo. However, in both cities the numbers are small.

Table 5.17 Entered hospital when referred – total sample (%)

	Nantong		Zibo	
	Entered hospital (%)	Number of referrals	Entered hospital (%)	Number of referrals
Timely	64	150	67	51
Other	35	26	63	30
All	60	176	65	81

Conclusions

Perhaps the most important conclusion that can be drawn from this study is that diversity is the primary characteristic of work unit-based urban health insurance in China. Attempting a simple description or, more seriously, proposing simplistic policy solutions is to disregard this simple fact.

That diversity has a number of related aspects. One is in terms of the need for health services. A number of the relatively new, often joint-venture, enterprises are predominantly staffed by young, healthy women. For most, there is little need for health care and the cost of provision is of marginal concern to their employers. Indeed, the only major requirement for many will be at the time of childbirth, and the one-child policy ensures that the cost implications of this are also strictly limited. At the other extreme are some long established SOEs, with both a substantial proportion of their workforce aged over 45 and a large number of retired workers who retain entitlements to health care.

If those SOEs are loss-making, their employees are very likely to be in low income households, particularly if, as in Zibo, the general economic environment is poor. And the members of those poor households are considerably less likely to be in work units which have joined the new health insurance schemes. The general pattern is thus one in which those employees with the greatest need of health care are least able to pay for it themselves and least likely to belong to schemes which will offset the cost. This position is compounded by the fact that other household members may be in a similar situation. There is a clear tendency for households to be composed of members covered by similar health insurance schemes, perhaps reflecting the likelihood of marriage between members of the same or similar types of work unit.

The effective value of health insurance schemes depends not only on their stated policies but also on the degree to which they meet their obligations. In this regard, the general finding from this study was much as expected. Employees in profitable SOEs experience minimal difficulties in obtaining health care cost reimbursement. This is also true for employees of government agencies in the more prosperous Nantong, but markedly less so in Zibo, where two of the three agencies studied were said to delay payments, though none failed to do so eventually. Loss-making SOEs performed badly overall, though it was interesting to note that three of the six enterprises in Nantong and two of those in Zibo were seen as functioning well. One-third of our sample were reported to be failing to make payments by a substantial proportion of their employees. Again, the picture is one of diversity. An employee of an unprofitable SOE may well continue to receive expected health care benefits but faces a considerably increased likelihood of finding that they are not forthcoming.

There was no clear evidence of any strong link between category of work unit and employee expenditure on health care, even though the reimbursement rates varied widely. Expenditure on chronic care, for example, was somewhat higher in Zibo, even though in work units other than government agencies and profitable SOEs the majority of employees received no repayment. The position appears similar for those entering hospital following a referral, with no evidence of lower rates in the less prosperous Zibo. However, the position is complicated by the fact that referral rates are themselves almost twice as high in Nantong. This may indicate that referrals are made partly on the basis of a patient's health insurance or personal financial position.

If schemes reported as providing timely reimbursement are compared with those which are not, there does appear to be some indication in Nantong that utilization rates are substantially higher for the former than the latter. This applies both to seeking treatment for acute illnesses and to hospitalization. In Zibo, the position is much less certain and the interpretation is difficult. Both incomes and reimbursement rates are low in Zibo, which may mean that even if covered by functioning health scheme, the co-payment required to enter hospital remains a substantial deterrent.

Overall, the impression is of a situation in which employees and households attempt to meet their health care needs either with or without the support of a good work unit-based insurance scheme. This has the implication that for poor households other consumption requirements may well be adversely affected. The correlation between ill-health, poverty and badly performing or inadequate insurance schemes may not provide an insuperable barrier to health care but does place yet another financial burden on a substantial number of poor employees and their households.

Chapter 6

Urban Health Reform in China: The Impact on Vulnerable Groups

Jiaying Chen, Henry Lucas and Youlong Gong

As discussed in Chapter 5, a majority of employed urban residents are members of work unit-based health care schemes, typically either GIS or LIS, and for this population the interest of the study was in the implications of the possible transfer of responsibility for their care to the new forms of HIS being implemented in each city. However, the research also wished to examine the position of those who might be in a less favourable position, with inadequate coverage by existing schemes and largely neglected by the proposed reforms.

This component of the study was conceptualized as relating to the problems confronted by various 'vulnerable groups' living within urban areas. Their common characteristic was to be that they were living in households with no member employed by one of the work units generally assumed to provide adequate health care coverage, namely government agencies, public institutions, SOEs or COEs. It was also intended that each group studied should be fairly narrowly defined, both in order to allow detailed exploration of the specific factors affecting their access to services and because the ultimate objective of the research was to propose possible policy interventions. As is well understood, one major concern when formulating such interventions is that they should be well targeted on the intended beneficiaries. Adopting definitions that could be used to readily identify individuals for the purposes of the research should allow for the possibility that similar definitions could be used by the authorities for effective targeting. As a first step in defining the groups to be selected for inclusion in the study, existing programmes which targeted such groups were considered.

Existing Programmes that Assist Urban Dwellers to Meet Health Care Costs

At present three distinct, though related, programmes exist that provide selected urban populations with assistance in meeting health care costs. The corresponding targeting mechanisms may be characterized as based on employment, income-poverty and 'vulnerability'.

The guiding principle of urban welfare provision in China from 1949 onwards was guaranteed employment and a package of work unit-based social benefits which included health care, education, housing and pensions. One component of the economic reform programme has been a move to transfer the social responsibilities of work units to municipality-based social insurance schemes, funded by contributions from employers and employees. Transition to the new systems is under way but taking longer than planned, partly owing to unexpected financing and management problems. Loss-making work units have sometimes been unable to join simply because they were unable to fund contributions. Current and former employees of profitable work units that have joined the new schemes are concerned that they provide somewhat lower benefits than their previous LIS. Special arrangements have had to be introduced for the increasing number of laid-off workers (*xiagang*). These can in theory receive a basic subsistence allowance and payment of contributions to pensions, health and social insurance schemes. However, the number receiving their full entitlement appears to be very limited (Cook, 2001).

For those identified by local officials as living in poverty or extreme poverty households, temporary financial relief (*shehui jiuji*) is available. The escalating number of laid-off workers and the movement of large numbers of the rural poor to more prosperous urban areas in search of higher incomes have contributed to a rapid growth in the number of the urban poor (UNDP and ILO, 2000). The number below the official poverty line is 13 million or some 3.5 per cent of the urban population (Hussain, 2000). However, Guan (1999) regards this estimate as very conservative and suggests that the figure could be as high as 15 per cent. In addition to the problem of income-poverty, there has also been a rapid rise in the number of urban dwellers without entitlements to social benefits such as education, health care and pensions. This is the position of the great majority of non-residents but it may also be the case for many employees and pensioners where the responsible work unit can no longer meet its obligations.

Given the numbers involved and the total funding available, it is clear that only a tiny proportion will be recognized as qualifying for *shehui jiuji*. A recent government response has been the establishment in 1996 of the 'Minimum Living Security' (MLS – *zuidi shenghuo baozhang*) assistance programme, which aims to meet the basic subsistence needs of urban residents whose income falls below a local poverty line. At the end of 2000, around 3.3 million people were receiving MLS (Gao, 2000). It is intended that this should rise to some 15 million, or 4–5 per cent of the total urban population (Tang *et al.*, 2000). However, when most household members do not have a regular source of income it is extremely difficult to develop an objective targeting mechanism and there are concerns that access to this benefit will often depend on the subjective judgement of local committees. It should also be noted that non-residents, in particular members of the floating migrant population, have no entitlement.

Finally, there are long-established programmes for the sustained support (*shehui fuli*) of vulnerable groups. These are sometimes identified as those who have no ability to work, no family and no source of income. It would include, for example, orphan children and the elderly or disabled with no families. Such people have traditionally been granted financial assistance from the state to meet their subsistence requirements. The identification of vulnerable groups and the level of assistance have been seen as questions best left to the judgement of local officials.

There are no official definitions of vulnerability and no national policy on the nature and extent of the assistance which should be provided for specific vulnerable groups. This is very much in line with the general tendency for decentralized decision-making on social policy issues. Again, the number of *shehui fuli* beneficiaries is relatively limited (Wu, 2003).

Review of the Chinese Literature on Vulnerable Groups

The next stage of the research involved a review of the Chinese literature on vulnerability and heath in urban areas. The aim was to explore which groups were most commonly identified in this literature.

As might be expected, a considerable number of authors (for example, Xu *et al.*, 1999; Liang, 1999) discuss the problems of the 'official' urban poor, those recognized as in need of financial support by responsible authorities. For this population, the rapidly escalating cost of health care is seen as a particular burden, given that they are already recognized as having great difficulty in coping with the routine expenditures required to meet their essential needs. In recent years much attention has also been directed at the households of laid-off workers (Cook and Jolly, 2001; Chen and Guo, 2000). Though formally retaining rights to work-unit health care and other benefits, the loss-making enterprises in which they were employed are typically unable to provide them with more than a small monthly payment which is far too little to meet the cost of services. There is also some evidence (Zhang *et al.*, 1999) that the health, and especially the psychological health, of this population is adversely affected by the stress caused by their radically worsened situation. Their need for services may thus be increased just at the time when their access to services is drastically constrained.

The nature and implications of the floating population, the prodigious number of migrants who have left rural areas in an attempt to share in the rapid economic growth that has transformed many urban areas, has attracted the attention of both policy-makers and academics in China. A number of studies have focused on the lack of entitlements to social services, including health and education, suffered by many members of this population (Ma, 2000; Wang *et al.*, 2000; Tian *et al.*, 1999; Zhan *et al.*, 2002). A key issue identified by these studies is the need to differentiate carefully between various types of migrant. The concerns of single men with pre-arranged, fixed-term employment, for example in the construction sector, are very different from those of migrant households, possibly with young children, whose main or only source of income is derived from selling fruit and vegetables in a local market.

As in many other countries, the provision of health care for the growing proportion of elderly people is a major and growing problem in China. Many studies have demonstrated that though they have high levels of utilization of services, this still underestimates their true need, given a reluctance (typically based on cost) to always seek care when required (Ou and Zhu, 2000; Zhou and Wang, 1998). This is of particular concern in relation to in-patient referrals, which are frequently not pursued. Populations with somewhat similar problems, in that health care costs constitute a major and long-term component of their routine expenditures, are the physically and mentally handicapped, the disabled, and the chronically sick (Wu *et al.*, 1999). For these populations much of the literature emphasizes the wide variation in the type and seriousness of the conditions suffered by individuals classified under these broad headings and the consequent need for policies which address specific needs.

Methodology

Based on the above, and in consultation with the city authorities, the following four groups were selected for in-depth research under the vulnerable groups component of the overall study:

1. Laid-off and unemployed worker households   Laid-off and unemployed households were defined as those in which a laid-off or unemployed member was the primary income earner. In Nantong they were sampled from the name lists of local street committees. In Zibo the households sampled were those whose main earner had a certificate of laid-off work or unemployment and were receiving regular subsidy from the municipal Bureau of Labour and Social Security. Some of these households were identified through street committees, but most were approached through the Bureau. Most of these workers were still covered by the LIS of their previous work unit, or the recently established HIS of the municipality, if their erstwhile employer had joined. In the former case, the LIS would assist with health costs if the enterprise was not bankrupt. In the latter, the Bureau would take responsibility.

2. Elderly households   Elderly households were designated as those where all adult members were at least 60 years old. However, during the fieldwork it was found that a limited number of selected households had another 'temporary' member, who was often said to be visiting to provide assistance. In Nantong many elderly households contained retired workers who were still entitled to support from their work-unit LIS. Some were in so-called 'special groups', including employees or cadre members who started work before 1949 and disabled ex-servicemen. These could obtain 100 per cent reimbursement of their health care. In Zibo, where urbanization was relatively recent, there were many 'neighbourhood commissions' (*juweihui*) based on former villages. Where these had some economic resources, they typically provided a retirement income of some CNY400 to CNY500 per month to elderly households. Most of the elderly had no health scheme coverage, though they might be given some subsidy for large expenditures.

3. Poor households   In Nantong the poor households sampled were selected from those designated by local agencies, for example the Bureau of Civil Affairs or municipal Labour Union. These households were eligible for limited financial support from these agencies. Many of those supported by the Bureau were elderly or widowed. They could obtain reasonably generous subsidies for their living and health expenses. Other households received regular welfare payments but no specific help with health care costs. Those designated by the Labour Union were mainly laid-off or unemployed workers whose enterprise had become unprofitable or bankrupt. They had no routine income or health care support.

In Zibo only a very small number of households were officially defined as poor by authorized agencies. Here poor households were sampled from a list based on the assessments of local street committees and neighbourhood commissions. Because these households were not legally designated, many did not receive routine payments from local government. Some obtained limited support from their neighbourhood commissions where these had income from collective enterprises.

4. Migrant households In Nantong migrant households were identified from the registration lists in two local police agencies. The households selected were those in which a family group had migrated. They included some households consisting of two or more adults, with and without children, and some in which a woman with children had travelled without her husband. Most adults were relatively young and healthy, and some were well educated with reasonable employment prospects. In Zibo the nature of the households was similar, but because of the absence of an effective registration system most were sampled in the marketplaces where they worked.

A district cluster sample of 500 households was selected for a community-based household survey in each city. These were distributed across the four identified sub-populations (laid-off/unemployed, elderly, poor and rural migrant), with 200 migrant households sampled and 100 households from each of the other groups. Street committees assisted in the identification of the four types of household in the districts selected for the survey.

Findings

Household Characteristics

The health status and health-seeking behaviour of households is dependent on their socio-economic status. Three specific factors are considered here: the age and sex composition and household income status.

Table 6.1 shows the age composition of each type of household in each city. Note that the 'elderly' households in both cities, contrary to the above definition, contain a substantial proportion of adult members under the age of 60. In most cases these were described as 'visitors' who were staying for varying periods of time with their elderly relatives, either to provide assistance or because they needed accommodation in that part of the city. It is also evident that in Nantong a considerable proportion of those officially classified as members of poor households are over the age of 60. A much smaller proportion of the members of laid-off worker households and a very small number of those in the floating population fall into this age band.

Table 6.1 Household type by age composition (%)

Household type	Nantong			Zibo		
	0–14	15–59	60+	0–14	15–59	60+
Laid-off	16	73	11	17	78	5
Elderly	5	12	83	4	16	80
Poor	9	52	39	12	60	27
Floating	21	75	4	17	82	1

Table 6.2 similarly provides information on the household sex composition. The most notable feature is the higher proportion of women in poor households in both cities.

Table 6.2 Household type by sex composition (%)

Household type	Nantong		Zibo	
	Male	Female	Male	Female
Laid-off	47	53	50	50
Elderly	47	53	48	52
Poor	39	61	44	56
Floating	50	50	50	50

Table 6.3 provides details on the economic status of the different household groups with reference to the national poverty line (PL) of CNY195 per month per capita. In Nantong the incomes of the elderly and floating population households are considerably higher than those of the other two groups. Around 86 per cent of members of the elderly and 68 per cent of the floating population are in households with per capita incomes more than twice the poverty line. Indeed, less than 4 per cent of members of elderly households are living below the poverty line. Laid-off households have around 7 per cent of members in poverty, similar to the figure for those in the floating population, though a further 63 per cent are in the next lowest income category. Note that around 10 per cent of members of the 'poor' households sample are in households with per capita incomes that are more than twice the poverty line. As discussed above, in Nantong these are households that were designated as poor by local agencies. The apparent contradiction may be due to a misclassification or it may simply be that the situation of some households has improved considerably since the original designation was made.

Table 6.3 Household type by poverty status (%)

Household type	Nantong			Zibo		
	<PL	<2PL	>2PL	<PL	<2PL	>2PL
Laid-off	7	63	30	7	53	40
Elderly	4	9	87	17	34	49
Poor	64	27	10	56	40	4
Floating	7	25	68	7	36	57

In general, the incomes of all household groups in Zibo tend to be below those in Nantong. This is particularly true of the members of elderly households. Some 17 per cent of these are in households with incomes below the poverty line and 51 per cent in households with incomes less than twice the poverty line. The poor households sampled in Zibo have very low incomes, with 56 per cent of members being in households with incomes below the poverty line and less than 5 per cent in households with incomes more than twice this value. Relatively few laid-off households fall below the poverty line, but a majority are in households which fall into the next income band. Again, the floating population households have somewhat higher incomes, with 57 per cent of members in households with incomes more than twice the poverty line.

Table 6.4 considers directly the extent to which the vulnerable group classifications overlap. Not surprisingly, the most important intersection relates to poor households. In Nantong some 42 per cent of these would also be classified as elderly and 21 per cent as laid-off, whereas in Zibo the comparable proportions are 23 per cent and 47 per cent. Again, the impact on poverty of failing SOEs is very evident in Zibo, whereas the official 'poor household' designation in Nantong is closely linked to the aged population even though, as indicated above, this appears to contradict their reported household income status.

Table 6.4 Cross-classification of household types (%)

Household	Nantong				Zibo			
type	Laid-off	Elderly	Poor	Floating	Laid-off	Elderly	Poor	Floating
Laid-off	–	0	0	0	–	1	0	2
Elderly	0	–	0	2	3	–	0	0
Poor	21	42	–	0	47	23	–	1
Floating	5	2	0	–	13	1	0	–

Sources of Finance for Health Care

Table 6.5 Health scheme coverage by household type (%)

Scheme	Nantong				Zibo			
	Laid-off	Elderly	Poor	Floating	Laid-off	Elderly	Poor	Floating
GIS/HIS	10	42	6	4	4	8	5	1
LIS	49	44	29	9	38	23	15	7
Other	15	7	14	5	9	8	6	3
None	26	8	51	81	49	61	74	89
Sample size	356	246	238	571	388	224	277	519

Table 6.5 indicates a possible reason for the relatively high income reported by the elderly households in Nantong, with 86 per cent reporting coverage by GIS/HIS or LIS, an indication of effective support from their former work unit. It also shows the great variation in health scheme coverage both between the sampled household

groups and between the cities. Overall, those in Nantong clearly have considerably better health benefits than those in Zibo. However the floating population and poor households fare badly in both cities.

Health Care Needs

Acute illness
As might be expected, the rates of acute illness shown in Table 6.6 are highest in elderly households. They are not much lower among members of poor households, although this can be at least partly explained by the prevalence of older people in designated poor households. The link between age and acute illness is also evident in the low rates for members of the floating population households. Figure 6.1 plots trends of episode rates by age and type of household. It can be seen that the episode rate increases with age in all types of household, and is typically highest across age bands in poor households and lowest in floating population households. This would correspond to an assumption that the circumstances of those in poorer households tend to make them somewhat more prone to acute illnesses, while those who have decided to migrate in search of an improved standard of living may be self-selected to be in more robust health. Note that migrant households in Zibo had lower episode rates than in Nantong in all age bands. This may be due to the method used to identify floating population members.

Table 6.6 Reported illness episode during two-week period by household type

Household type	Nantong		Zibo	
	Patients per 100	Episodes per 100	Patients per 100	Episodes per 100
Laid-off	25	29	16	19
Elderly	44	57	42	50
Poor	37	53	33	40
Floating	18	19	8	9

Chronic illness
Table 6.7 shows that in Nantong members of elderly and poor households also report very high chronic illness morbidity rates, with almost 50 per cent of the elderly suffering from such an illness and 44 per cent of the poor. Again, the rate for poor households is almost certainly a reflection of their age structure. Overall, around 56 per cent of those over 60 reported some form of chronic illness. The members of the floating population households, with very few members aged 60 or over, again report the lowest rates, with a prevalence of less than 9 per cent. The situation in Zibo is similar but again influenced by the lower correlation in this city between the poor and elderly household classifications. Overall, poor household members reported a chronic illness prevalence of 33 per cent, while those over 60 reported 70 per cent, even higher than in Nantong. The rate for the floating population households is just 4 per cent, half that in Nantong. However, the numbers involved are insufficient to draw any conclusions.

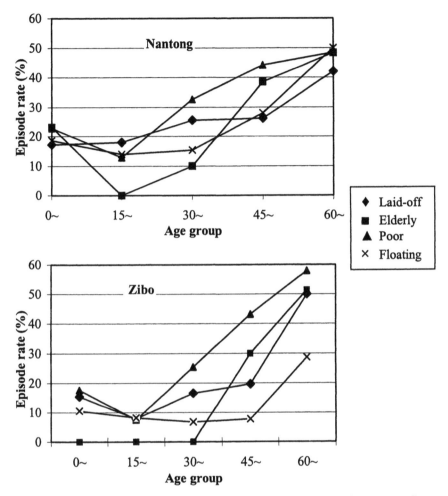

Figure 6.1 Episode rates by household type and age group in Nantong and Zibo

Table 6.7 Prevalence of chronic illness by household type

Household type	Nantong		Zibo	
	Illness rate (%)	Illness rate (% of ≥60)	Illness rate (%)	Illness rate (% of ≥60)
Laid-off	19	50	10	50
Elderly	50	57	50	59
Poor	44	57	34	70
Floating	9	*	4	*

*The number of members in this category is too small for sensible comparison.

Hospital referral

The final indicator of health care need is provided by the number of household members referred for in-patient treatment (Table 6.8). Members of elderly and poor households have considerably higher rates than the other household types, in both cases mainly due to their age composition. Overall, some 57 per cent of all referrals in Nantong and 52 per cent in Zibo are for those over the age of 60.

Table 6.8 Hospital referrals by household type

Household type	Nantong		Zibo	
	Members referred (%)	Referrals per 100 persons	Members referred (%)	Referrals per 100 persons
Laid-off	5	6	4	5
Elderly	16	21	12	14
Poor	10	11	14	18
Floating	3	4	2	2

Health Services Utilization

Acute illness

Table 6.9 shows the out-patient care utilization rate for reported illnesses over a two-week period. In Nantong members of the elderly households have by far the highest such rate. This may partly reflect the perceived severity of illness but is probably also strongly influenced by the high level of GIS/HIS coverage for this group. Overall, those in the GIS/HIS in Nantong have utilization rates twice those in LIS schemes and three times those paying out of pocket. In Zibo most utilization rates are considerably higher than in Nantong and the distribution across the household types varies considerably. Contrary to the pattern in Nantong, migrants report the highest rate (58 per cent) and those in elderly households, in this case without the benefit of GIS/HIS support, the lowest (24 per cent).

Table 6.9 Use of facility over a two-week period by household type

Household type	Nantong			Zibo		
	Visit rate by patients (%)	Visits per 100 people	Visits per year per capita	Visit rate by patients (%)	Visits per 100 people	Visits per year per capita
Laid-off	18	7	1.9	35	7	1.7
Elderly	32	20	5.1	24	28	7.2
Poor	14	8	2.2	36	18	4.7
Floating	18	4	1.1	58	5	1.4

The higher utilization rates for three of the household types in Zibo probably reflect the lower cost of services. As discussed above, whereas in Nantong care is typically provided by hospital out-patient departments, many patients in Zibo will make use of lower level enterprise or private clinics. Given that the members of all vulnerable household categories in Zibo and all but members of elderly households in Nantong typically have to meet health care costs by out-of-pocket payments, it is not surprising that utilization appears to be closely related to cost. On this basis, the high utilization rate for migrants in Zibo may relate to their relatively high income levels and infrequent need for services. Note that the elderly in both Nantong and Zibo, because of their high level of reported need for services, have the highest estimated number of visits per year per capita. Their annual cost of treatment is thus likely to be considerably higher than for other groups.

As might be expected, the most frequently stated reason for not using services was that the illness was 'not serious'. However, it should be noted that in Nantong the proportion in this category was considerably lower for household members covered by GIS/HIS. It seems plausible that this indicates an indirect effect of treatment cost, with household members being more inclined to treat acute illnesses as less serious if the out-of-pocket cost is high. Cost was the second most important reason given by all household members in the two cities for not seeking care.

Chronic illness
The great majority of those reporting chronic illness also indicated that they had sought and received medical assistance. Some 90 per cent of those in poor households, the least likely to seek advice, had received a formal diagnosis and of the 88 per cent who were then prescribed treatment almost 80 per cent said they were following that prescription (Table 6.10). There is some evidence that the failure to treat chronic illness is influenced by cost. Among those with no insurance in Nantong some 25 per cent were not following their prescription as compared with just 10 per cent who were covered. However, this may also relate to the actual or perceived severity of the illness, given that the latter group includes many of those in elderly households.

Table 6.10 Diagnosis and treatment of chronic illness by household type

Household type	Diagnosed (%)	Prescribed (% diagnosed)	Taking treatment (% prescribed)
Nantong			
Laid-off	99	88	97
Elderly	98	96	90
Poor	91	88	⤴ 79
Floating	94	83	85
Zibo			
Laid-off	95	87	91
Elderly	96	94	98
Poor	89	89	87
Floating	100	89	94

In-patient care
Overall in Nantong around 56 per cent of those referred to hospital were admitted. Members of elderly households were most likely to go into hospital, again probably reflecting both the greater seriousness of illness and superior health benefits available for this group. Differences between other household types were limited and probably not significant, given the small numbers involved. In Zibo poor family members were least likely to go into hospital, with an admittance rate of less than 45 per cent compared with around 70 per cent for other groups. This would seem to reinforce the impression that the ability to pay for services is a key factor in Zibo, given the relatively limited importance of the various health insurance schemes for these household groups.

Health Expenditures

The overall economic burden of health care
Health expenditures over the previous two weeks were used to estimate an annual total. This was then added to the cost of in-patient services over the previous year to derive an estimate of annual health expenditure. The total expenditure and out-of-pocket component are shown by household types in Figure 6.2, which also provides estimates of the latter as a proportion of household income per capita. Overall, the total costs for laid-off and floating households are relatively low in both cities, while for elderly and poor families they are extremely high, particularly in Nantong. However, as would be expected, out-of-pocket expenditure is considerably higher in Zibo for all groups. Those in poor households in both cities have the highest economic burden, spending almost 17 per cent of per capita household income on health care in Nantong and around 28 per cent in Zibo. The contrasting position of the elderly in the two cities is clearly demonstrated by the 6 per cent of per capita household income paid by those in elderly households in Nantong compared to the 20 per cent paid in Zibo.

The cost of chronic illness
The various health care schemes tend not to provide special reimbursement arrangements for most chronic illnesses. Even in the relatively well-funded HIS in Nantong, for example, just six chronic conditions are identified for special consideration. Patients claim for out-patient visits in the same way as for acute episodes. However, as chronic illnesses may require frequent out-patient visits and long-term treatment regimes, cumulative expenditure can be very large and, even with apparently generous reimbursement, may entail considerable out-of-pocket payments.

Expenditures for members of different household types suffering from chronic illness in Nantong and Zibo are shown in Figure 6.3. Again, total expenditure, the out-of pocket component and expenditure as a proportion of per capita household income are illustrated. Overall in Nantong the average self-payment per illness is CNY808, or 12 per cent of the annual per capita household income. This reflects the fact that most chronic patients are in the elderly and poor households. While the cost per illness is higher for the former group, CNY2,950 for the elderly and

CNY2,585 for the poor, their out-of-pocket payments are much less, CNY555 and CNY1,234 respectively, amounting to 6 per cent of annual per capita income for the elderly household as compared to nearly 45 per cent for those in poor households. The floating population also pay around two-thirds of the cost of treatment out of pocket, though on average this amounts to just 8 per cent of their relatively high incomes.

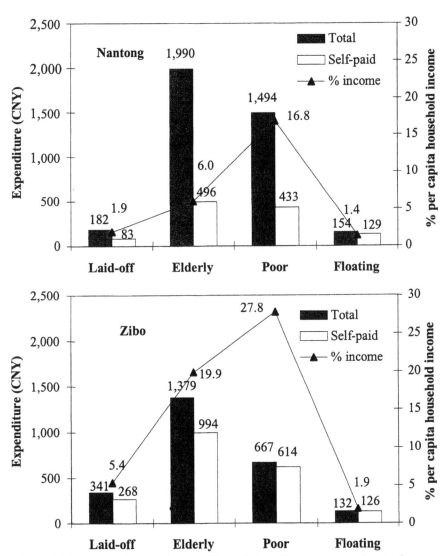

Figure 6.2 Estimated annual expenditure for health services and out-of pocket expenditure as per cent of per capita household income

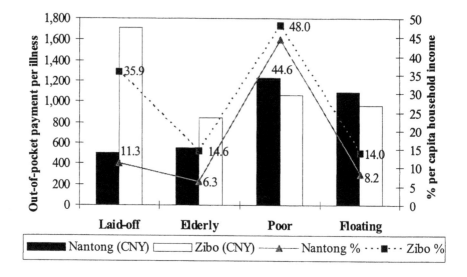

Figure 6.3 Out-of-pocket payment per year for one illness and as per cent of household per capita income in the two cities

As discussed above, the cost of health services in Zibo is generally below that in Nantong. However, lower incomes combined with lower reimbursement rates mean that the average out-of-pocket expenditure for chronic illness is around 23 per cent of per capita household income, almost twice as high as that in Nantong. The pattern across household types is similar. Expenditure on each chronic illness for members of poor households is almost 48 per cent of per capita income. Very little of the total cost is reimbursed. Laid-off workers have the highest reimbursement (nearly half of expenditure), but on average they also spend the largest amount per illness and their out-of-pocket costs amount to some 36 per cent of per capita income.

Conclusions

Perhaps one of the most important findings of this component of the study relates to the difficulties encountered in simply identifying members of the specified vulnerable groups of household. Both approaches to identifying poor households, but particularly the adoption of the official designation in Nantong, resulted in samples which included a significant proportion of the less poor. The identification of elderly households, formally defined as those with no adult member under 60, failed to exclude those in which a younger relative was visiting, often on a long-term basis. Some households where the main income earner was a laid-off or unemployed worker retained LIS support for health care costs, while others did not. These targeting issues arose in a situation in which research teams were attempting to apply carefully considered definitions. In any official scheme aimed at providing assistance to such groups it is likely that the problems of correct identification will be much greater.

The study also clearly demonstrates the extent to which the defined vulnerable groups had different health care needs, levels of access to services and costs. It is evident that a one-size-fits-all approach to providing assistance would almost certainly be highly inefficient in terms of resource allocation. The elderly households in both cities face serious problems in having to meet the cost of chronic and in-patient care. However, in Nantong the burden is considerably eased by existing support systems, which appear to provide reasonable incomes and levels of reimbursement. As elsewhere in China (Zhan *et al.*, 2002; State Council of China, 2000), the floating population households in both cities have almost no access to health insurance schemes but generally have some of the highest income levels and lowest needs for heath care. The urgent need for this group would seem to be for some form of 'catastrophic' health insurance to address the very small risk that a serious health condition prevents them from working for an extended period.

The comparison between Nantong and Zibo raises interesting insights into the importance of considering both demand- and supply-side issues and their interaction. Nantong illustrates the possibility of achieving high levels of insurance scheme coverage among certain groups and in particular appears to protect the elderly reasonably well. However, the high cost of treatment, which may well be linked to the success of these schemes, means that those without coverage bear a very heavy financial burden. Though income levels, health insurance coverage and reimbursement rates are all low in Zibo, the situation appears to be at least sustainable because the nature of the supply side results in health care costs which are relatively affordable.

There was strong evidence of a high correlation between poverty and ill-health. In both cities, members of elderly and poor households reported markedly higher rates of acute illness. Overall, the rates were 40 per cent for those in elderly and 34 per cent for those in poor households. However, all age-specific rates were higher for the latter group. Prevalence rates of chronic illness follow the same pattern, with 50 per cent of elderly household members and 40 per cent of poor household members reporting chronic illnesses. Again, age-specific rates were uniformly higher for the poor. In line with results from other studies (e.g. Oxaal and Cook, 1998), poverty is also seen to reduce access to health services, with utilization rates considerably lower than for other household groups. For illnesses reported to need treatment, cost was given as the most important barrier to health service. In addition, there was some evidence that potential cost also played a role in determining when illness was regarded as sufficiently serious for treatment to be required.

Much has been written on the links between catastrophic illness and poverty (e.g. Asian Development Bank, 1999; Leon *et al.*, 2001). However, for many more households chronic illness is a major factor in the inability to move out of poverty. The impact may involve not only long-term expenditure on treatment and medicines but also a loss of productive capacity for both the individual concerned and those in the household who provide care. While the study did not gather data on these opportunity costs, direct out-of-pocket expenditure on treatment for chronic illness in Nantong and Zibo were found to account for a high proportion of household income. In poor households it amounted to 45 per cent and 48 per cent respectively of annual per capita household income. Most health schemes in China, including those in Nantong and Zibo, do not provide special reimbursement for chronic illness. This is against a background of population ageing and epidemiological transition. Cancer, cerebro-vascular disease and heart disease are the most important causes of death in urban China, accounting for over 85 per cent of the total in 1997 (Yang, Y., 1999). Assisting those with chronic health problems to cope with the resultant economic burden must be a major concern for policy-makers involved in the design of health insurance schemes.

The minority of households in the sample with reasonable health scheme entitlements were much more likely to use services. This is most clearly shown by the elderly households in Nantong, whose utilization of services and out-of-pocket expenditure was substantially reduced because of higher health benefits. The establishment of schemes designed to meet the needs of specific vulnerable groups that could provide equivalent benefits for all urban residents would clearly make a considerable difference to their well-being.

Chapter 7

Health and Vulnerability

Thomas Uhlemann and Fei Yan

The combination of general societal developments in China and the dysfunction of various systems (such as the health system) jeopardize the security of the entire population. However, not all strata of society are affected equally. The increasing dissolution of state and publicly funded health care has placed certain population groups in an especially precarious position, putting wide sections of the population at risk of impoverishment.

This problem becomes evident when normal day-to-day living is aggravated by illness or loss of a source of income. The interdependence of illness and the social system is often evident in these cases. The familiar vicious circle of illness and poverty – illness can cause poverty and vice versa – hits the poor particularly hard, when, as with a large portion of the unemployed or with the 'floating' population, no health insurance protection is available. The GIS and LIS have not been effective in addressing the issue of equity in access to health services for these groups. Approximately 40 per cent of the entire urban population of China is uninsured (Ministry of Health, 1998b, p.18).

Health insurance is of little use when employees are unable to secure reimbursement – as in the case of poorly managed or money-losing enterprises. It is now apparent that it was a mistake not to establish some kind of risk pooling across enterprises or across local and regional governments. For people whose lifestyle was already limited, unemployment or a further deterioration in health could lead to a life-threatening crisis. Chronic illness or a physical disability result in constant monetary difficulties due to the costs of medicine and treatment which run parallel with a diminished ability to work.

The new health insurance programmes are, like GIS and LIS, strongly oriented towards the average urban employee. Businesses and their staff are in the front line of the state's attempt at insurance reform (Ensor, 1999). It was therefore assumed that not all segments of the population would profit from the health reforms evenly; specifically it was accepted that there would be certain segments of society whose entry into the health service plan would be limited for different and varying reasons. The recognition of the life situations of these segments of society would seem to suggest the concept of 'vulnerability'.[1] Cook (2001) describes the new forms of vulnerability as an expression of the economic and social revolutions in Chinese society:

While many have benefited from new economical opportunities and higher incomes, new forms of risk and vulnerability now face certain population groups, particularly those falling outside the urban employment-welfare system. At the same time, a significant number of people remain in chronic and absolute poverty, marginalized from the processes of growth and market development (Cook, 2001, p.3).

Changing Patterns of Vulnerability

After examination of the literature and discussion with official representatives from politics, administration and health care institutions, it was possible to identify population groups which were particularly vulnerable with regard to adequate health care provision. This applies in particular to the following five urban population groups (defined in the Annex):

- The unemployed and laid-off workers.
- People with disabilities. Some have normal or casual work, some stay at home or even need daily care by a family member.
- The elderly. Some have good pensions and health insurance, some have pensions but no health insurance, while some have neither pension nor health insurance.
- Rural-to-urban Chinese migrants. Some are well off because they have good businesses whilst others struggle for survival.
- The poor – recipients of social support financed by the Ministry of Civil Affairs.

With the reform of many systems, especially of enterprises, the gap widens between health needs of the vulnerable and their ability to access health care. In addition, the number of the vulnerable has gradually increased, most noticeably the elderly, poor and disabled groups but the laid-off and migrant vulnerable groups are also increasing. The incomes of the vulnerable are very low and increase at a slower rate than the average while current medical costs are comparatively high. Poverty leading to sickness and sickness leading to poverty is a serious problem.

There have been only a few studies of the living conditions and health of these groups. Liu and MacKellar (2001) looked at the challenges faced in the areas of old-age pensions, health care and disability services. From their point of view, demographic changes make some increases in spending inevitable, although they do not suggest how to finance such needs. Others (Liu *et al.*, 1999; Li, 1999) tried to evaluate the pilot reform in Zhengjiang City with regard to its effect on certain groups of the population. Krieg and Schädler (1995) described the framework and conditions of the new social security system (*shehui baozhang*) and the situation of underprivileged groups.

The situation of these segments of society did not noticeably improve after the health insurance reforms at the end of the 1990s. In addition, many improvements have remained only 'on paper'. The realization and execution of the new reforms often means certain groups are unable to filter through the system to make official health claims. Even though the new scheme provides some protection for the elderly, the degree of protection is often marginal and rarely more than modest. As for migrant workers and the poor, they were not covered nor the aim of the reforms.

The aim of this qualitative in-depth study of two cities, Nantong and Zibo, was to identify life situations and health opportunities for those with limited or no insurance cover, and to describe to what extent existing institutions and health services are used by vulnerable groups.

How Vulnerable Households Cope with Health Problems: Nantong and Zibo

This section presents the results of the studies of vulnerable families from Nantong and Zibo. We focus on the whole group in both cities; differentiation of the individual segments within the whole group or between the cities is only made if there is a special quality in the difference.

Socio-economic Situation of the Samples

In total, 65 households (including a number of pilot interviews) were interviewed, 33 in Nantong and 32 in Zibo. The interviewees were equally divided between female and male. The interviewees consisted of the following five groups: laid-off workers/the unemployed, the disabled, the poor, the elderly and migrant workers. The transitions between these groups were fluid and permeable, for example, several unemployed households could also be categorized as poor. So the segments into which the households have been divided are meant for analytical purposes: 12 households belonged to the migrant workers group, 12 to the disabled group, 13 to the laid-off/unemployed group,[2] 14 to the poor, and 14 to the elderly group. The average age of the interviewees was 56.1 years. The migrant workers were the youngest of the groups with an average age of around 38.5 years. The size of the households varied between one and six people. The poor had the smallest and the disabled group had the largest average number of members.

Income and its main sources

The households included in the survey were predominantly poor, that is, the average income was in the lower tier of urban households. The definition of poverty varies from city to city; According to Mr Shen, Director of Social Security of the Municipal Workers' Union, on 10 August 2000, in Zibo the Civil Affairs Bureau paid CNY143 per person per month as relief for the disabled and poor and the Labour and Social Security Bureau paid CNY130–180 to unemployed and laid-off workers. In Nantong the Civil Affairs Bureau usually paid CNY156 per person for the poor and disabled by of local government, but poor people over 60 years could get CNY180 a month, while the disabled might get less than CNY156 if their family conditions were not so poor. The laid-off and unemployed group received CNY195 a month from the Labour and Social Security Bureau. This situation is mirrored in the selection of the sample and poverty was a significant selection criterion.

The monthly family income ranged from CNY96 to CNY40,000. The migrant group had on average the highest (CNY760 in Nantong, CNY384 in Zibo) and the poor had the lowest (CNY187 in Nantong, CNY178 in Zibo). Between that the average monthly income per person of the disabled was CNY248 (Nantong) and CNY186 (Zibo), the elderly CNY754 (Nantong) and CNY323 (Zibo), and the laid-off/unemployed CNY360 (Nantong) and CNY355 (Zibo) (see Table 7.1).

The main sources of incomes were salaried jobs, pensions, business and various types of social relief. Income sources were specific to the different groups: whilst, depending on their status, elderly people lived mostly on their pensions (usually paid by companies) and migrant workers tended to be dependent on 'work on the move' (construction sites, etc.), the other three groups of society received their incomes from a mixture of sources. Laid-off and unemployed workers and the disabled supported themselves from a mixed bag of pensions, social relief, work on the side and other small jobs. The poor we interviewed received state support but most were also supported by their social network.

Table 7.1 Monthly income and its source in Nantong and Zibo

	Nantong average monthly income (CNY)	Zibo average monthly income (CNY)	First source of income	Second source of income
Migrants	760	384	Casual work	Own business
Laid-off/ unemployed	360	355	Subsidy	Casual work
Elderly	754	323	Pension	–
Disabled	248	186	Social relief	Odd jobs
Poor	187	178	Social relief	–

Apart from migrant workers, who generally sent money to their relatives in the countryside, almost all the members of the other groups could only afford major or unexpected expenditure by receiving money from relatives. Such expenditure could be due as much to illness as to a family celebration such as a wedding.

A further characteristic was the irregularity of the household income. Alongside a relatively stable income, additional sources would become available only sporadically. These included, in order of importance, support from relatives, occasional work and one-off payments from firms, institutions and administrative authorities. Furthermore, self-employment income was sometimes seasonally affected. The amount of orders for small service industries and the turnover of convenience stores were also tied to seasons or festivities such as the Spring Festival. Income fluctuations of up to 30 per cent were not uncommon.

Expenditure and its structure

The largest expenditure (50 per cent of total income) was for food, followed by health at 30 per cent, with the remaining 20 per cent covering costs such as rent, services (e.g. electricity, gas and water), telephone and housing. This division of income was comparatively inflexible, with hardly any opportunity to alter the expenditure breakdown. Correspondingly, apart from the migrant households, very few households were able to save for special occasions or later purchases. Expenditure for clothing was not significant, as many families would go for many years without buying new clothes, wearing hand-me-downs from relatives or neighbours.

These proportions do not give any indication of the actual level of expenditure. The fact that 50 per cent of the income was spent on food reflects the poverty of these people: meat and fish hardly ever appeared on the menu, which consisted predominantly of rice, oil and vegetables. These basic nutritional supplies were not always sufficient, which is why gifts from the stores of the local authorities on special occasions such as the Spring Festival included rice and oil.

Broadly speaking, the monthly level of expenditure for most of the families was matched by the income. The income of the poor and some unemployed and elderly was not sufficient to cover all the normal costs, and so these groups had to depend on loans from friends and relatives. Although repayment was promised, the families of very limited means simply could not do so. Borrowing money actually means asking for a contribution, which everybody knows cannot be paid back. Only the migrant worker families were able to save money. The saving quota was normally 10–15 per cent of the net income. This money was saved mainly in order to support relatives who lived in the countryside or (in Zibo) to buy a house near their place of work.

Housing and other facilities

A large proportion of the families interviewed lived in their own flat or house; renting was not common. On the one hand, not having to pay rent is a considerable relief for many households but, on the other hand, the purchase of a flat or house is an expense that leads to voluntary debt. Money can be borrowed from relatives and, less commonly, from firms.

The average number of rooms (excluding kitchen, which often was not in a separate room, but including bedrooms) was three. The average flat size was 54 m^2 for an average household with three members. This results in an average 20 m^2 per person. There was a correlation between the income and the fixtures and fittings within the flats. A lower standard would commonly include no electrical appliances apart from, for example, an old, second-hand black and white television. There would be nowhere for visitors to sit and clothes would be stored in plastic bags rather than wardrobes. There was comparatively little space for members of the floating population since they tended to live in small flats or houses or in a small area in their business such as a shop. A higher standard would include a colour television, refrigerator, washing machine, telephone and air-conditioning. The description and self-evaluation of their living conditions was based extensively on the existence of the technical equipment described above.

In general the existing housing conditions of those interviewed as part of this study were no reason for concern or causing particular problems. While some families from the migrants group were planning to purchase a house or flat, others did not regard it as necessary since they had come from another area where they owned a house to which they would return in due course. However, it must be pointed out that the circumstances of the families interviewed did not necessarily cover the entire spectrum of possible conditions of life. It is certain that extreme conditions are only portrayed as an exception. Due to the form of the sampling, certain groups were not covered, including a not inconsiderable population of migrants who work illegally and have no permanent place of residence. Such people often drift from construction site to construction site, using the sites as sleeping areas, sheltered by cardboard. The word 'residence' cannot be used in this context.

Health Insurance

Exactly half of the interviewees and their families in Zibo and one-third of the Nantong families had absolutely no health care cover. In 30 further households only one member was covered, in two households two out of three members had insurance. In only one household (two pensioners) were both members completely covered.

There was a tendency for the pensioners and the laid-off and unemployed workers to be better covered than the migrants, the disabled and the poor. Many of the insured were forced to wait for a long time until their claims were accepted and reimbursed, and there was often uncertainty whether the company responsible at the time was even able to cover the claim. Often businesses refused to pay their contributions to the system, arguing that they were having financial problems of their own and so could not afford to pay.[3] Some of the interviewees blamed the uncertainties of the law in this area.

The security of these 'insured' households was, at best, mostly limited to in-patient treatment and care, or it was limited by percentage of coverage or an upper limit of reimbursement. In addition, in many cases there were special regulations and uncertainties. It is evident that households which were unable to save money for such situations found themselves in a serious financial predicament due to the delay in reimbursement from companies. In very few cases did the health insurance protection completely cover all costs. Almost all the interviewees had to pay the additional costs themselves. Because of their general exclusion from most of the benefits that town-dwellers receive, migrants and the poor had to pay all medical expenses from their own pockets; it was usual for them to ask the providers (hospitals, doctors) for a discount. In many cases the payments and the contributions of the Labour Bureau for Unemployed took on the character of charity, which appeared to depend on the good will of the participating authorities.

All in all, households cannot calculate their expenditure on health; they are not able to make plans for unforeseen expenditure. Attempts at saving money by cutting down on personal expenditure for health will always be undermined by recurring crises in their health situation. Possible savings will be exhausted by treatment very quickly. If the financial resources of a household are not sufficient, money will be borrowed from relatives or, in the case of migrants, from friends to cover costs.

Use of Health Services

Health status and perceived health problems

Nearly 70 per cent of the interviewees suffered seriously from at least one chronic illness, which made it necessary to have a constant supply of medicine. The following illnesses were noted among the interviewees (in the order of their occurrence, from the most frequent to the least): bronchitis, stomach problems, high or low blood pressure, diabetes and various heart ailments. Some of the interviewees attributed their illness and the difficulty of being cured to their circumstances, for example, the condition of their apartment. Above all, lung diseases, which could be attributed to air pollution and problems in heating, could become chronic.

A closer view of the under-insured households shows that health deterioration was especially likely if families were faced with in-patient treatment and unavoidable expenditure for pharmaceuticals on an unexpected scale. In these situations the ability of the families to pay was exceeded very quickly and they tried to move the boundary between illness and ailment in favour of ailment. This led them to substitute expensive drugs with self-treatment and household remedies such as relatively cheap herbs and traditional medicine. Patients sometimes did not buy or take drugs prescribed during or after out-patient or in-patient treatment because the prices were not acceptable for their families. Pharmacies that were integrated into hospitals were especially unpopular because of their high pricing policies.

The utilization of health services was definitely correlated with the financial well-being of the interviewees: treatment or purchase of medication occurred only if insurance existed or a significant reimbursement could be expected.

Access to health services

Hospitalization Hospital care was avoided as much as possible, for admission was mostly bound up with costs which the interviewees could not afford. The deposit for hospital admission, alone, which is, with the exception of emergency cases, around CNY1,000 in some hospitals in Zibo, prevented admission, according to some interviewees. Hospitals in Nantong and Zibo reported that the proportion of in-patients who suffered from minor diseases was less than the proportion suffering from serious diseases.

Despite considerable health problems very few of the interviewees had been admitted to hospital in the past few years. The people who were self-financing specifically avoided out-patient care and in-patient treatment, as the registration fee was charged regardless of the severity of the illness and prescription drugs were expensive in the hospital. Most patients wanted to leave a hospital as soon as possible and asked the doctors to discharge them. Over 80 per cent of the in-patients of the Zibo Central Hospital in 2000 wanted to be discharged as early as possible to minimize costs. An exception was the pensioners who were in possession of a medical card that guaranteed them free care or a large proportion of reimbursement. This group frequented medical clinics of all types (and at all levels) considerably more often than all the other interviewees, even for mild illness; moreover, a visit to the doctor was more usual and caused less concern about payment.

Out-patient visits Out-patient care through hospitals and clinics was used more often by people who had insurance than by the uninsured. However, here also possible costs of treatment by a doctor were weighed against the possibility of self-treatment through the advice of a pharmacist and buying the medicine themselves.

Because of their multi-morbidity and their relatively good health insurance cover, elderly pensioners were over-represented in doctor visits. They frequented the out-patient clinics often or regularly. Migrants who were self-employed visited the doctors the least. As a group they were comparatively healthy and at the same time shrank from spending money on medicine. The time spent at the doctor played an important role with migrants. Several of the interviewees said they would not be able to close their business temporarily or let somebody run it while they were away, without being afraid of losing money. Contract workers feared losing their jobs.

It was not said directly, but some of the interviewees gave the impression that sometimes the insurance of a single member of a family was used to acquire treatment or drugs for other family members. Appointments with doctors or clinics were made under the name of the insured family member.

Choice of health institution The choice of a hospital or clinic depended on the type of insurance held. The insurance given through their workplace usually bound people to specific institutions. According to the type of illness the interviewees were referred to a specialist or to a better-equipped hospital. If a specific hospital or clinic was not written into the insurance policy, the insured person could chose a clinic in his or her area or according to personal contacts. Perhaps a relative worked in a hospital as a nurse, a neighbour was a doorman in a clinic, etc. This considerably eased entry into hospital and care. The medical equipment and the specialization of the hospital or clinic was as a rule of no concern to the interviewees and so was not a criterion in their choice.

Coping with sickness – unmet health needs
More than half of the respondents had unmet health needs. This applied especially to the poor and the disabled group, but also to the elderly and laid-off respondents without health insurance or low reimbursement rates (see Box 7.1) and to a few of the floating migrant group. Most unmet health needs were of a minor nature; those with colds, dizziness or backache would not go to a hospital. However, they sometimes failed to attend hospital in the case of a serious disease. A few respondents admitted that they had been advised to be hospitalized by a doctor but had not complied. Others did not visit a doctor because their health insurance

package had a limited percentage of reimbursement or a fixed amount a month (laid-off workers received subsidies of CNY10–20 a month; some interviewees received CNY30 a month or CNY200 a year), or because their work unit was a loss-making enterprise and delayed reimbursement.

Box 7.1 Examples of vulnerable groups with unmet health needs

Ms Gu (disabled group, blind, chronic nephritis): 'When we have a cold, usually we do not go to see a doctor, we just have more boiling water.'

Ms Zhou (laid-off group, hurt leg in car accident): 'I was asked to go to hospital, but I did not comply. The doctor asked me to have surgery to remove the metal plate. It will cost CNY3,000. It is impossible for me to spend such a lot of money.'

Mr Yi (poverty group, no health insurance): 'My feet cannot be radically cured. The medical cost is so expensive, I cannot afford it, so I just buy some liniment to embrocate my feet sometimes.'

Mr Zhong (elderly group, Parkinson's disease); his wife said: 'His medicine has to be saved, because he just has CNY50 a month to be reimbursed. If his disease is stable with no attacks he will not go to hospital and I go to the hospital to get medicine for him. Because if he went to hospital they would want to hospitalize him, but he would not comply. He took three tablets three times a day when he was hospitalized before. After his discharge he just took one or two tablets a day usually and when he shook seriously he took a few more tablets. He begrudges the use of the medicine because of the cost.'

Health conduct always goes hand in hand with lifestyle, which is determined by various factors, such as socialization, work and living conditions, social relationships and the local structure of health services and what they offer. There were different reactions to illness; there were also different coping habits. Behaviour during illness, such as seeing a doctor, buying medicine from a pharmacy, asking insured family members to obtain medicine from a doctor, obtaining assistance from others or using local/natural remedies, depends on various factors.

Nearly all interviewees differentiated between an ailment, which did not require a visit to a doctor or could be cured with over-the-counter medicine, and illness. The impression is that the differentiation varied according to the wealth and the perceived severity of the illness. If illness made treatment or a hospital stay necessary, the perception of the illness and compliance depended directly on the financial situation of the patient. Symptoms were reinterpreted and therapies were very often left unfinished, resulting in the disease becoming chronic.

The decision-making algorithm in Figure 7.1, from perceiving the symptoms to self-treatment, help through the lay system or the use of professional medical treatment, was determined in many ways by the personal situation and the social climate. Influencing factors included: type and range of expected costs; size of the expected reimbursement; coverage of the health insurance; financial possibilities;

support from friends and relatives; experience with the illness; and basic knowledge of possibilities of cures. With this background the severity of the disease was determined and a decision made whether and which help was needed.

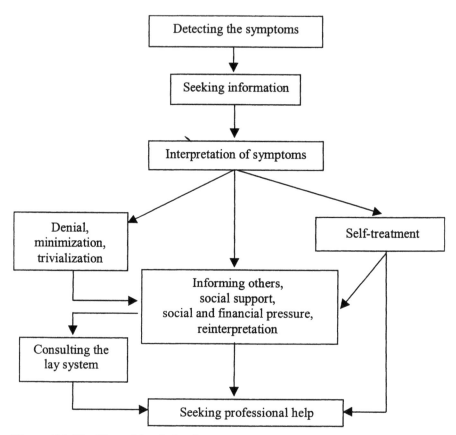

Figure 7.1 Health-seeking behaviour

It is possible to identify in principle three solutions for coping with illness: first, decide to do nothing and wait; second, self-treatment; and third, try to get professional help. How families decide is above all dependent on whether they have insurance or not. If the sick person is insured, or at least someone in the family is insured, then he or she usually chooses to go to a hospital. If there is no health insurance, then the decision whether to wait and see or to start self-treatment rather than seek professional help is dependent not only on the financial capability of the family but also on the social environment and the personal disposition of the person involved.

The influence of the social context can lead to reinterpretation of the illness. Within this is also the so-called lay system, in which non-professional experience is sought. Decision-making processes are established in which self-treatment, lay-system experience and professional help will be given a different position of importance each time.

Medical Costs and Their Financing

The average expense for the treatment of illness ranged from CNY50 to CNY4,000 per year. The absolute limit of expenditure was determined by whether in-patient care was needed or not. Chronic or acute illnesses had a little more influence on the decision. Between the individual segments of society there were considerable differences and families of old-age pensioners in particular had to pay.

The average total out-patient medical expense for a family was around CNY600 a year. There were some differences between the groups. Most of the elderly families spent CNY200–900 a year for their health. Three of the poor families spent less than CNY100 a year. The out-patient medical expenses of other families in this group ranged between CNY100 and CNY1,000. Most of the disabled families spent less than CNY500 a year on out-patient medical care although the highest medical expense of all groups (CNY3,400) was incurred by a disabled family. Laid-off families spent between CNY200 and CNY1,600 a year. Most floating families spent CNY500 a year. Very few families spent more than CNY1,000 a year on out-patient medical costs and very few had no costs.

More important than the absolute limit of expenditure was the share of the health costs which had to be paid out of pocket from household income. In extreme cases almost 50 per cent of the total income of a poor family had to be used. On average the poor families paid the absolute smallest amounts, but the share of these costs of their total household income was higher than for any other group (25–40 per cent). The migrants had to spend on average a somewhat higher sum, but the share of the household income was merely around 6 per cent. The households of the poor tended to spend little on medical costs because they simply lived with illness or cope with it in other ways. The medical costs were low in comparison to those of other groups, around CNY200–1,000 a year, but it was a comparatively large expenditure for them and impacted a great deal on their daily lives. Some asked for help from relatives, friends, neighbours or neighbourhood or street committees in the form of medicine or loans.

The main ways to finance medical costs were:

• Payment by health insurance. Regardless of the kind of health insurance or the percentage of reimbursement, respondents who had health insurance would receive reimbursement and the remainder would be paid out of pocket. As mentioned before, some interviewees had to wait to obtain reimbursement because their unit's profit margin was poor.
• Via household members' health insurance. In some families, a member who had health insurance obtained medicine from a hospital or clinic and gave it to a member without health insurance.
• Getting help from others. Some respondents said their medicine was donated by their children, relatives or friends.

Social Support

The interviewed families relied on a wide range of social support. Comparable to findings reported in the literature (Cook, 2001) the interviewed families primarily relied on safety nets provided by people close to them. Informal support was predominantly given by relatives, neighbours, (former) colleagues or friends. The floating population were again an exception. Their relatives still lived in the countryside and therefore they relied on help from other groups and friends. Support mostly came for specific items, such as purchasing a flat or house, and for unexpected expenses such as treatment in hospitals, operations or the purchase of medication. Guaranteed repayment was rarely given and was not really expected in the foreseeable future.

It is uncertain if families in the future will be able to maintain their function within social networks, because there is a tendency towards the nuclear family. Increasingly, the younger people wish to live separate from the old generation – an aspect of the modern world that China faces like other countries.

Depending on their responsibility and ability to help different institutions could be consulted as part of formal, government-regulated social support. Sometimes applications for support were refused if there was any indication of other support, for example from relatives. The authorities seemed to have considerable flexibility in their management and a lot of freedom in their decision-making processes. The Zibo Municipal Health Bureau agreed with health service providers a small discount of around 10 per cent for the medical care of the poor. It was up to the health facilities to apply for this discount on behalf of the patients.

Concerns About Health Insurance and Services in the Future

Almost all respondents worried about health care costs in the future, especially the elderly and poor groups. They said that they could always eat and dress simply, but they would have no way of covering the expenses needed to treat a serious disease. Hence, they sincerely hoped that the government would propose a special health insurance scheme for them.

The main concerns and fears regarding future problems and difficulties seemed to vary depending on age. Among the younger interviewees the economically tense situation led predominantly to depression and fatalism ('we will wait and see' or 'one shouldn't really waste too many thoughts on this'), whilst among the middle-aged wishes and worries related more to their children's education and their house and home. The older population, however, clearly feared that they would no longer be able to manage and maintain the fragile balance of their everyday lives and health. This balance and the future wishes of the middle-aged were mostly threatened by possible illness or the worsening of existing illnesses and the resulting costs for treatment and medication. This prospect was so threatening because, as mentioned above, the cost of health insurance was usually not affordable.

Comparison of Nantong and Zibo

The initial key finding was the comparatively low quality of life in the selected households in both cities. The average income of a vulnerable household was significantly below the average income of the populations of Nantong and Zibo (around CNY447 for the urban in Zibo and CNY222 for the rural population) and also below the average income of the Chinese urban population. In both cities a large number of households were supported by the Civil Affairs Bureau, Labour Bureau, street committee, neighbourhood committee, other family members, relatives, friends and neighbours. The family was the most common source of support for the vulnerable households. The health conditions of the samples in the two cities were quite similar.

There were, however, obvious differences between the income of the groups in Nantong and Zibo. Generally, the income in Nantong was significantly higher. There was only a little difference in the income range within the groups. Housing in Zibo appeared to be better and cheaper than in Nantong; the flats and houses were relatively bigger and newer in Zibo. Fewer laid-off people had a contact with the Labour Bureau in Zibo; the subsidy in Zibo (CNY130–180 a month) was lower than in Nantong (CNY195 a month). The living standard in general appeared lower in Zibo.

More disabled and poor people received relief from the Civil Affairs Bureau in Nantong (three out of six disabled, six out of seven poor) than in Zibo (two out of six disabled, four out of seven poor). The relief from the Civil Affairs Bureau was greater in Nantong than in Zibo. In Nantong disabled and poor people received CNY156 a month with poor people aged over 60 receiving CNY180 a month, whereas in Zibo the rate was CNY143 a month for disabled and poor people. There was also more help from society for vulnerable people in Nantong than in Zibo. Some organizations such as banks and youth unions donated money or goods to poverty or disabled people.

On health matters, people in Zibo visited community clinics or health stations more often, while people in Nantong more often visited hospitals or unit clinics. More people in Zibo had experience of not using health services when they were sick. The percentage of medical cost compared to income in Zibo was a little higher than in Nantong.

Existing Provisions to Support Vulnerable Households

The two cities have had various policies, regulations and spontaneous actions for supporting vulnerable people:

- Providing the so-called 'five items insurance' (food, clothes, living, medical services and funeral expenses) for the elderly without any income or child;
- Providing monthly relief to those without any income, without people to be dependent on and without working ability, and to the families of old disabled soldiers, elderly veterans and old martyrs;

- Setting up a minimum living standards line and giving monthly relief to the people below that line;
- Donating some part of the lottery funds to a social welfare fund to support services to the elderly;
- Support from society, for instance, donations from various enterprises, public agencies, private companies or individuals and daily help from neighbourhood and community volunteers;
- Several pilot community health service stations to improve the vulnerable's access to health services.

Conclusions

Good health for the urban population is not unified. Certain groups are considerably more disadvantaged and have less chance of good health care than the average citizen. Good health in the long run (health opportunities) is to be understood as a combination of environment, such as work and living conditions, the individual's health habits, for example exercise and tobacco use, and the ability to take advantage of the health care system. The sub-study presented here aimed to bring into focus several of these conditions.

The period during which this study was executed marked concurrent fundamental changes in the social security system in China. In this connection the investigation of especially vulnerable households played a considerable role in the reform of health insurance (that is, the transition from the GIS and LIS system to the new basic health insurance scheme). Officially, that means the system gives a new series of advantages to pensioners, the disabled and legal migrants. Other groups, such as the poor and illegal migrants will not take part or will be given only a very small role in the reform. Specific additional reforms, for example, the setting up of a medical help fund for the poor, are only being planned or are currently still under discussion.

At the time of the implementation of this study the reforms had not yet had any effect on the interviewees of the vulnerable households. The entry of the interviewees into the health services was for various reason extremely limited and it is assumed that this situation will continue, as an expansion of state maintenance of the health care system is not intended.

Reasons for the perpetuation of an extremely desolate situation lies above all in the very limited financial means of the individual households, which cease urgently needed treatment, mainly in-patient hospital care, because they cannot afford the registration fees. In the face of this financial shortfall, serious diseases are reinterpreted so that the families rationalize self-treatment or waiting in the hope of spontaneous healing. This often results in the disease becoming chronic and the suffering not only weighs down the individual household, but also the health care management system with further and higher costs.

Starting programmes to work against this development lie on one hand in improved health care education (above all for migrants) and on the other hand in additional state or municipal programmes for the coverage of health costs, especially for the poor. Finally, the creation of strong competition between the health care providers could also lead to an easing of the situation. This would demand a policy which would make economic reserves of the existing system available to the vulnerable households. Developing community health services would increase availability and accessibility for the vulnerable, and decrease the gap between their health needs and utilization.

Notes

1   The concept of vulnerability corresponds to the sociological concept of 'social situation in life' (*Lebenslage*), which attempts to encompass inequity as a complex 'happening' or 'event' in which quasi-natural characteristics such as sex, age and ethnic group are combined with economic determining factors and opportunities of participation. The aim of the concept is to depict an actual situation in life and to uncover the factors that contribute to a deprived social situation.
2   It was estimated by the Zibo Municipal Government that the number of laid-off workers was around 30,000. Representatives from the Women's Federation reported an estimated number of roughly 100,000 laid-off workers. The official unemployment rate in 2000 is 3.4 per cent.
3   There was some evidence for this argument. Zibo with its old heavy industries was faced by an economic depression and for an increasing number of (especially state-owned) enterprises it was becoming increasingly difficult to cover the health costs of their employees and retirees.

Chapter 8

Gendered Impacts and Implications of Health Sector Reform in the Context of Multiple Transitions in Urban China

Rachel Tolhurst, Hilary Standing and Xu Qian

Urban China is currently undergoing profound economic, social and demographic transitions. Gender is an important factor in the uneven effects of this transition on individuals and households. Gender is critical to social policy because it underlies the social division of labour and the returns to labour in terms of economic and social benefits. It associates 'reproductive' work – the tasks associated with child-rearing and care-taking in the household – with women, and simultaneously allocates lower social and economic returns to this work. Changes in the organization of labour and its returns are central to China's transition. The gender division of labour, and associated beliefs about the capacities and roles of women and men, shape the responses of individuals, households and institutions to the transition to a market economy. For example, evidence is emerging of changes in participation by different groups of women in 'productive', or income-earning, work, and consequently their access to the social and economic benefits of such work. Gender also interacts with, and is qualified by, age and cohort. Age interacts with gender to affect the ordering of productive and non-productive activity over a person's lifetime, for example through time taken off work because of childbearing. Finally, in addition to age, cohort is particularly significant in shaping an individual's position in social relations and labour markets, especially where major transitions have occurred or are occurring over people's lifetimes. For example, the educational levels and work histories of women in China reflect to a considerable extent the historical period in which they came of age (Rofel, 1999).

This chapter focuses on health care as an important social benefit that has been affected by the current transition. The ongoing reform of public institutions and state-owned enterprises in urban China has had a profound impact on the financing, organization and provision of health services. This has raised major concerns about increasing inequities in access to health care. We introduce a framework for analysing the impact of economic liberalization and health sector reform on different groups of women and men in urban China, using findings from the studies reported in this book, and discuss the implications for health reforms and social security.

Gendered Impacts of Economic Liberalization and Health Sector Reforms

Impacts of Economic Liberalization on Women's Position in the Workforce

We will begin by briefly outlining trends concerning the position of women within the workforce. Significant gains were made since the founding of the People's Republic of China in gender equality in the workforce, through legislation to protect women from discrimination and propaganda campaigns promoting women's role in production.[1] However, some areas of production retained a high degree of gender segregation and those enterprises which employed predominantly women, such as collectives, offered lower pay and benefits (All China Women's Federation, 1991; Druschel, 1999). In addition, it has been argued that the nature of the work unit (*gonzuo danwei*), which was the basic building block of urban Chinese society under communism, played a significant part in gender equality gains after 1949. This was because it took a great degree of responsibility for areas of workers' lives designated by Western capitalism as part of the reproductive sphere, such as child care, housing and health care, thus enabling women's participation in the labour force on more equal terms with men (Stockman, 1994).

The economic transition is, however, bringing about changes in women's position and opportunities in the workforce. Liberalization has led to a number of policy changes to increase competitiveness of state-owned enterprises. Work unit managers have been able to use redundancies, 'early retirement', transfers and leave with basic pay to meet the new demands on enterprises (Howell, 1997). The development of new types of enterprise, including joint ventures, and the market reorientation of older enterprises, has led to the demand for new skills amongst workers (such as marketing, sales, accounting and computer skills) and preferences for particular types of workers. There is mounting evidence that managers making human resources decisions in this new market environment refer to gender and age stereotypes in deciding which kind of workers to hire and fire. For instance, there is a bias in redundancy against women, especially older women (Cook and White, 1998). Female redundancies may also be hidden in forced 'early retirement', which is permissible earlier for women than men (as early as 35 in some cases), and in other categories such as 'maternity leave'[2] (China Rights Forum, 1998) and there is some evidence of an increase in the gender ratio amongst early retirees (Standing, 2001). There is also some evidence that women find it more difficult to get reemployed than men[3] (Gustafsson and Li, 2000).

Young, unmarried women are likely to be the preferred employees of foreign-investment enterprises, but older married women are increasingly discriminated against, partly because enterprises wish to avoid the costs of providing women's health benefits such as maternity leave and insurance coverage, and breast-feeding time. Almost 70 per cent of enterprise managers interviewed in Shenyang and Nantong indicated a preference for employing men and 30 per cent of leaders stated that they wished to recruit only men (Howell, 1997). This discrimination extends to professional women (Davin, 1990; Druschel, 1999).[4] Rural women migrants without support structures or legal residence are especially vulnerable to abuses of their rights as workers. Jobs taken on by rural migrant women tend to be highly marginal, temporary and unlikely to include social security benefits (Feng, 1997).[5]

There is a continuing and widening wage gap between women and men, which varies between different economic sectors and by cohort and age (Standing, 2001). Estimates of the gap vary widely between 42 per cent (Maurer-Fazio *et al.*, 1999) and 84.4 per cent (Gustafsson and Li, 2000). The causes of the gender gap are debated, and may reflect labour market segmentation, with women more likely to cluster in lower paying enterprises, gender differences in educational levels, and gender bias in the allocation of benefits such as overtime (Standing, 2001). Since urban pension levels are determined by years of service, lower retirement ages for women also mean that they receive lower salaries and sometimes reduced benefits.[6] Laid-off women have also been found to receive lower pay packets than laid-off men[7] (China Rights Forum, 1998). Das Gupta *et al.* (2000) argue that for some women increasing gender gaps in wages have cause a marked drop in family and social status and have led to changes in bargaining positions and decision-making power in some households.

A growing proportion of the urban population, such as the unemployed and economic migrants without city residence permits, are not eligible for any employment-related benefits, or they are entitled to further reduced benefits, such as those on short-term or temporary contracts and those who have been laid off or 'early retired'. Even the reduced benefits offered to laid-off or 'early retired' workers may not be paid (China Rights Forum, 1998). This process does not directly discriminate against women – there is no evidence that there is any difference between the insurance benefits given to women and men within enterprises. However, if women are over-represented in those groups that are vulnerable to benefits cuts or losses, such as those working in loss-making enterprises, those laid-off or 'early retired' or those unemployed, this constitutes an indirect bias against women in the distribution of benefits. Additionally the majority of dependants received some benefits under the previous system but these benefits have now been substantially reduced. As we argue in the next section, social, demographic and epidemiological transitions are likely to combine with labour market changes to put increasing pressure on women to focus on child-rearing and care-taking roles. If this is the case, the erosion of benefits for dependants will also disproportionately affect them.

Other Changes: Social, Demographic and Epidemiological

The above major changes in the labour and benefits systems have been developing at the same time as other major changes in the structure of urban Chinese society and trends in health and health care. First, as discussed elsewhere in this volume, there has been a rapid escalation of costs of health care. This trend has coincided with reduced benefits coverage to threaten the affordability of health care for a number of groups. Second, China is undergoing a demographic transition to an 'ageing society' as a result of a decreasing rate of population growth due to the one-child policy and an increase in life expectancy. Third, urban China is passing through a 'health transition' from an epidemiological profile in which communicable diseases featured prominently to one in which the main burden of ill-health is due to non-communicable diseases. Fourth, the liberalization of the media in China has also changed public discourse on the roles of women. Since 1949 state social engineering projects have used mass communication to espouse the emancipation of women, laying emphasis on women's social and intellectual equality with men and their importance as workers to the success of the task of socialist construction.

A number of commentators have discussed the new social discourses which are appearing and which, rather than extolling the heroic woman worker of socialist iconography, see her as increasingly 'unproductive,' of 'poor quality' (less educated or skilled) and unable to adapt to the changing needs of the labour market. Women who were earlier seen as full economic and social citizens now find themselves part of the socially excluded (Cook and Jolly, 2001; Rofel, 1999; Das Gupta *et al.*, 2000). At the same time, younger cohorts of women are increasingly defining themselves – or having their identities defined – in more 'feminine' terms (Rofel, 1999). This feeds a growing discourse which contradicts the official discourse of gender equality but is consonant with the ways in which the labour market is being restructured, with more clearly delineated 'women's jobs' and sectors emerging. As unemployment rises, calls to give preference to male job seekers are also increasingly being heard. Urban China may be witnessing a return to more traditional views of women's role in society and in the division of labour within the family (Milwertz, 1997).

These three changes are intersecting with changes in employment and benefits to produce a different environment for women both within and outside the family. The combination of the demographic shift to an ageing population and the epidemiological transition to non-communicable diseases will produce an increasingly heavy burden of chronic diseases, particularly amongst the elderly, with an increasing ratio of elderly dependants with chronic diseases to younger workers and carers. This dependency ratio will increasingly raise questions about how health care for the elderly will be financed. In the current environment women are likely to face pressures from both societal and familial expectations that they will take on the majority of the care associated with this disease burden. This in turn raises questions about the implications for the status and social security entitlements of carers, which will have particular relevance for women.

Gendered Vulnerabilities and Health Sector Reforms

An Analytical Framework for Understanding Gender, Age and Cohort in Urban China[8]

Rapid transition, of the kind being experienced in China, is having complex and difficult to predict effects on vulnerabilities. This framework is an attempt to capture some of these complexities in terms of likely emerging and cross-cutting vulnerabilities. The main purpose of the framework is to move analysis of the social sector away from a focus on fixed, vulnerable groups towards a more dynamic understanding of vulnerability. It is important to stress that not all women and not all elderly people are vulnerable. It is more useful to think of vulnerability as a dynamic process, rather than as a fixed property of certain groups. It arises out of particular combinations of attributes and social and historical processes. Gender and age combine with a range of external factors – economic, social and historical – to produce particular patterns of security or vulnerability. This is important from a policy perspective for two reasons. First, a preoccupation with fixed, aggregate groups such as migrants and the elderly runs the danger of focusing on groups that may not necessarily be at risk and missing groups which are less visible but with greater needs. Second, social sectors need to look ahead and identify emerging trends where action may be needed. The framework is very provisional. There are not sufficient data to substantiate some of these possible impacts. Equally, the complex and dynamic nature of the processes that produce vulnerability may mean that other configurations of gender, age and cohort will become significant.

Three vulnerabilities in urban China and their associated age, gender and cohort characteristics are explored here (see Table 8.1). *Asset vulnerability* refers not only to tangible assets, but also to human capital endowments, to social capital deriving from the networks which employment gives access to, and to family and kin-derived resources which are particularly significant to the non-employed. *Entitlement vulnerability* refers to the potential loss or reduction of benefits that derive from the state, employers or membership of a household with its associated entitlements. In relation to health care, health insurance is a key entitlement. *Social exclusion* refers to the ways in which poor and vulnerable people can find themselves outside the structures and institutions that provide opportunity and voice in society. These have a compounding effect on poverty and low status.

An individual's ability to meet the cost of health care depends on his or her entitlements or assets at the time of need. Entitlements and assets are accumulated over time, through serving in the workforce or for a particular work unit, earning a salary which enables the individual and other household members to save for a sufficient length of time, and raising a family, or nurturing family or social networks. Conversely, individuals and households can experience a series of events or processes that reduce their capacity to accumulate entitlements and assets over their lifetimes. These include: discontinuous employment (for example, in short-term or temporary contracts); redundancy; early retirement; low wages in relation to costs of living; changes in family composition; bereavement (death of wage-earning household members); ill-health, through the incapacity of the individual or other household members to work due to chronic illness; and depleted savings due to a high-cost episode or chronic illness. Gender, age and cohort influence the ability of individuals to accumulate assets and entitlements and their risk of failing to accumulate or losing them.

It is important to note that there is nothing intrinsic to women or elderly people that creates vulnerability to poverty or loss of entitlements. It arises from social and historical factors and circumstances. Women and elderly people who have been able to build up and hold onto an assets base will not experience any greater vulnerability unless this base is eroded by factors such as divorce or failure of a pension or other benefits scheme.

Table 8.1 Framework for analysing gender, age and cohort vulnerabilities in multiple transitions

Emerging vulnerabilities	Age/gender cohorts most affected	Asset vulnerability	Entitlement vulnerability	Social exclusion
Laid-off/ susceptible to be laid-off workers	Older SOE workers, particularly women.	Lower human capital endowments among 1950s generation. Loss of social capital, e.g. networks to help find new employment. Interrupted employment disrupts ability to save.	Loss of formal workplace-based entitlements in urban areas, such as health insurance and pension provision.	Age and gender discrimination in workplace leading to social discourse of 'low quality' people, negative effects on identity and self-esteem and loss of social networks.
Casual workers	Young male and female migrants from areas of high poverty. Older, less-educated workers.	Migrants' rural asset base likely to be limited. Low human capital endowments (e.g. education) limit employment prospects and wage levels. Interrupted employment disrupts ability to save.	Lack of or loss of formal workplace-based entitlements in urban areas, such as health insurance and pension provision.	Lack of 'citizenship' in urban areas leading to discrimination in entitlements and lack of access to formal institutions and legal redress.
Elderly non-employed lacking viable income	Laid-off/retired without pensions. Likely to be more women than men.	Capacity to access family/kin resources may be fragile due to changing family structures.	Lack of formal workplace-based entitlements in urban areas, such as health insurance and pension provision.	Social isolation.
Chronically sick/disabled and their carers	Elderly will preponderate among sick. Elderly women may be more vulnerable. Other female family members may be carers.	Capacity to access family/kin resources may be fragile due to changing family structures.	Lack of formal workplace-based entitlements in urban areas, such as health insurance and pension provision. Lack of entitlements to care.	Employment and social discrimination.

Methodological Issues

There has been little research into how gender influences access to health care for urban women and men. There are a number of methodological difficulties in researching the vulnerabilities discussed above in such a rapidly changing environment. First, as we suggest above, women as a group do not necessarily share common vulnerabilities. In survey research, therefore, simply disaggregating data by sex provides little evidence of vulnerability. Women may be particularly vulnerable within other identifiable vulnerable groups, such as the laid-off or the elderly, although again this is not necessarily the case. In a survey that aims to capture the general dimensions of vulnerability, such as the one conducted during this research, the sample size of each vulnerable group identified is often too small to enable meaningful comparisons of the situation and behaviour of women and men within these groups, especially where the differences between women and men are unlikely to be uniform.

Second, more sensitive indicators of vulnerability are needed which treat vulnerability as a dynamic process rather than as a fixed property of certain groups (Standing, 2001). The sub-study on vulnerable groups initially identified these as the poor (as designated by street committees), the elderly, the disabled, migrant workers and laid-off workers. However, the study suggests that whilst these are potential indicators of vulnerability for individuals because they represent some of the pathways to entitlements loss, they are not sufficiently sensitive (because many individuals in these groups have sufficient entitlements) and they are not comprehensive (in that they may miss individuals who have suffered a critical loss of or inability to accumulate entitlements over time). Additionally, because they are household-level indicators, they may not capture the gender-related vulnerability of individuals such as dependants and carers, who may suffer a loss of entitlements at an individual level.

Third, a cross-sectional survey cannot easily reveal trends in women's and men's situations and behaviour over time, and is therefore limited in its usefulness to capture the process and cumulative effects of broken career histories, for example. Longitudinal methods such as cohort studies may be more effective in tracing the emergence of vulnerability and identifying useful indicators.

Fourth, it is difficult to capture the dynamic and shifting nature of vulnerability and how gender interacts with age and cohort to shape this through single research encounters with individuals. Although qualitative research offers the advantage of providing an opportunity for the respondents to voice their own perceptions of their situations and positions, the very 'normalization' of gender roles and relations through ideological processes often acts to ensure that women (and men) do not perceive or articulate gendered disadvantage as such. It can therefore be difficult to ground an analysis of gendered differentiation in either empirical or subjective evidence. Longer-term engagement with women and men through qualitative and participatory research that offers opportunities for participants to reflect on their histories and experiences may help to address this problem. Bearing these limitations in mind, the following sections aim to provide some evidence, both qualitative and quantitative, of emerging gendered vulnerabilities, and suggest areas for further investigation.

Trends in Gender Differences in Health Insurance Entitlements

Health insurance coverage
The National Health Services Survey of 1998 found that a greater proportion of urban women than urban men had no insurance coverage, although the gender gap decreased between 1993 and 1998, suggesting that a greater proportion of men than women lost their insurance coverage during this period. The discrepancies in the proportion of women and men without health insurance across the income quintiles are shown in Table 8.2.

Table 8.2　Percentage of women and men with no health insurance in urban China by income group, 1998

Income group	Male	Female	95 CI%[9]
1 (Poorest)	70.51	74.21	1.10–1.32
2	52.45	59.19	1.22–1.42
3	39.53	46.68	1.28–1.50
4	31.01	34.69	1.10–1.28
5 (Richest)	24.14	24.81	0.95–1.13

Source: National Health Services Survey Data.[10]

It is likely that this difference in coverage between women and men reflects the proportion of women and men in full-time employment versus housework or retirement rather than differences in access to benefits within employment. It is also notable that, except for the poorest, the gap widens in the poorer quintiles.

In individual interviews with female and male workers, laid-off workers and retirees, few clear gender differences in the career histories of older working women and men emerged that might affect access to health care benefits. However, a number of young women workers interviewed who had short-term contracts or were laid off either had no health insurance or lost this when contracts ended. We have seen that women are represented disproportionately in some of these categories, which points to a potentially increasing source of disadvantage in health entitlements for these groups of women. Additionally, a number of older women interviewed had no benefits due to having been housewives or carers for most of their adult lives.

In the community-based survey described in the Annex a greater proportion of women than men in both cities paid for their own health care (i.e. had no health insurance). For example, 74 per cent of women in Zibo did not have insurance as compared to 62 per cent of men, whilst in Nantong the percentages were 48 per cent and 44 per cent respectively. However, this sample could not be generalised to the community.[11]

Insurance coverage for women's health services

It is important to give specific consideration to women's health, both because of its special emphasis on preventive care and because there is generally a relationship between the low status of women and lack of adequate provision for women's specific health care needs. Historically in the People's Republic of China women's health has been well protected and catered for by specific legislation and work-unit responsibilities. For example, the Female Workers Health Care Regulations state that women approaching menopause should receive gynaecological check-ups every one to two years (Article 13) and that all female workers should have fixed check-ups for gynaecological or breast conditions (Article 14). However, in the current situation, women without full employment (e.g. housewives, migrant women workers, unemployed women and some laid-off women) are unlikely to be offered any preventive services. In the community-based sample survey, 16 per cent of women in Nantong and 31 per cent in Zibo had received a women's health examination in the previous two years. Different types of enterprise also offer different levels of women's health care entitlements. The enterprise-based survey found that some types of enterprises were significantly more likely to offer preventive screening exams for women than others. For example, in Zibo 82 per cent of women working in a public institution and 81 per cent of women working in an SOE had been offered women's health preventive screening in the previous two years, in comparison to 60 per cent of women working for a private company and 58 per cent of women working in a collective enterprise. In Nantong 63 per cent of women working in a public institution and 46 per cent of women working in an SOE had been offered such screening, in comparison to 33 per cent of women working for a collective enterprise and 16 per cent of women working in the private sector.

Insurance coverage for maternity care

Another area where benefits are being eroded for certain groups of women is that of pregnancy and maternity benefits. Historically, maternity benefits (in both health care and leave) were enshrined in legislation. Work units are still required to provide maternity benefits by law and not to discriminate against pregnant women. However women workers on temporary or short-term contracts are vulnerable to effective dismissal if they become pregnant, because they have no maternity rights and employers are able simply not to renew their contracts. The 'one-off' nature of a birth in an urban household means that many households are able and willing to cater for the expense of the pregnancy and birth where public provision is not available. However, the sense of social exclusion suggested by the loss of benefits was keenly felt by one laid-off woman, who said. 'It's as if I don't have a connection with society'. The ability of families to absorb the costs of health care during maternity also depends to a certain extent on household entitlements such as savings or support from relatives. The story of one young mother suggests that where the lack of maternity benefits, coupled with the difficulty of finding work and childcare, coincide with unforeseen expenditure in the household this can lead to hardship:

A woman (29) had not been re-hired by the clothes factory where she had worked for two years three months after she became pregnant. At around the same time her mother-in-law became ill and needed care, so she did not look for another job. The costs of care for her mother-in-law's illness prevented the family saving any money for the baby. She chose not to stay in hospital after delivery to save money, but they still had to borrow about half of the cost of delivery from colleagues and friends, and later borrowed some more money for other expenses. They had managed to return some of the money, but were still in debt and planned to repay this when their situation improved. She said that they now needed to be very careful with their money. She planned to look for another job when the baby was eligible for kindergarten, but was not optimistic about getting one (Zibo).

Other studies have pointed to a particular concern with respect to the reproductive health of migrants, noting for instance the considerably lower take-up of ante-natal care among this group. Zhan *et al.* (2002) found that rural-to-urban migrant women made considerably fewer ante-natal care visits than permanent resident women in the Minhang District of Shanghai. Almost half of the migrant women giving birth at the three hospitals in Minhang district, during the period under review, did not attend any ante-natal care services during the pregnancy, contributing to the overall poorer outcomes for the migrant group. This was attributed to low rates of insurance coverage, low family incomes and low education amongst migrant women as compared to urban residents and to the low social status of migrant women, who felt marginalized and discriminated against by hospital staff.

Vulnerability of dependants to loss of formal entitlements
Dependants are also particularly vulnerable to the loss of entitlements. The example below illustrates how the death of a major family breadwinner led to the loss of indirect access to health care benefits at the same time as substantially reducing the resources available to the family to seek care.

A middle-aged widow lived with her mother-in-law, daughter, son, daughter-in-law and grandson. Only her son had full-time work. She had never had a formal job and stopped doing casual work to care for her husband. Whilst her husband was alive she received reimbursement for health care through his work unit when she asked the doctor to write his name on her prescription. Since her husband's death, all three of the women in the family including herself suffered from chronic health problems (including dizziness, swollen legs, heart problems, chronic pelvic inflammation and lung disease) but no one in the family ever visited the doctor because 'there is no money'. The family received CNY115 a month from her husband's work unit, but no other official relief (Nantong).

Trends in Gender Differences in Assets

A potential source of inequality in the individual's ability to pay out of pocket for health care or to accumulate savings to do so is the discrepancy in pay between women and men discussed above. Some studies conducted in urban China in the late 1980s and early 1990s suggest that households have generally pooled resources and that whilst there has been some variation in decision-making norms and patterns amongst urban Chinese couples and households, in most cases the woman has been responsible for the day-to-day management of resources, with the male 'head of household' being responsible only for occasional 'major' decisions such as investments (Whyte, 1984; Sha *et al.*, 1995; Zhang, 1994). In support of this, our qualitative interviews found that both women and men generally take for granted their right to use family resources to access health care and do so with little hesitation. However, Das Gupta *et al.* (2000) argue that for some women, increasing gender gaps in wages have cause a marked drop in family and social status and have led to changes in bargaining positions and decision-making power in some households. It will be important to conduct research to monitor this trend in the future. Our study also provided some examples of situations where particular women felt less entitlement to use family resources to access health care.

Several women interviewed had always been housewives and consequently had no health insurance or personal source of income or savings. Their husbands had pensions and some health insurance entitlement. Whilst all of them used health care in some form, they struggled to provide some contribution to the cost or they rationed their use of health care because of concerns about the cost, suggesting that they did not feel fully entitled to use health care because of their lack of financial contribution to the household. This 'self-rationing' of health care took an extreme form in the case of one elderly couple interviewed as part of the study of vulnerable groups:

> A woman of about 80, who had spent much of her life as a carer for her mother-in-law, was illiterate and had never had a job. Her husband needed full-time care for several severe chronic conditions. He had a pension and was entitled to health insurance but this was often delayed and was insufficient to meet the costs of his care, with the result that he reduced his medicine dosage. His wife suffered from a swollen face, hands and feet, and dizziness, but had not been to see a doctor. She said, 'I can only hope to serve my husband well. I hope I can die before him. I do not have labour insurance. I am willing to die before him. Only when he is alive, can I expect something. I feel very sad that I am not covered by labour insurance…[When I feel dizzy] sometimes I just lie in bed. If both of us take medicines we can't afford it.'(Nantong).

Individuals who are effectively dependent on their families, such as widows who never had stable formal employment and therefore no pension, may not qualify for state assistance because of the ability of the family to support them. However their dependent position may lead to a feeling of reduced moral entitlement to care, as is suggested by the following example:

> A widow of 73 lived on her own. She had been a carer for her mother-in-law since 1963. She received a small state subsidy and regular financial support from her two children, who both had financial problems themselves. Her children paid for any hospital visits or medication but she generally avoided using medical care for acute or chronic illness. She could not get any help from the Civil Affairs Bureau or Street Committee because 'they say I have a son and a daughter. I do not belong to those who can get any help from the government.' Her only wish was that 'I have no illness. I cannot afford to be ill.' (Zibo).

Although the numbers are very small, the vulnerable groups survey also provides some indication that older women are less likely than older men to seek health care for recent illness. In both cities, a smaller proportion of women over 60 sought care for self-reported illness. In the Nantong community survey, 19 per cent of women over 60 sought care for self-reported illness in the last two weeks, in comparison to 34 per cent of men and 19.6 per cent of all women sought care in comparison to 27.8 per cent of all men. In the Zibo community survey, 33 per cent of women over 60 sought care for self-reported illness in the last two weeks in comparison to 40 per cent of men, and 29.7 per cent of all women sought care in comparison to 33.3 per cent of all men.

Implications of the Transition for Future Gendered Entitlements

The gender differences in the capacity of an individual to accumulate formal and familial entitlements to enable them to meet the costs of health care may widen in the context of the major social and economic changes described in the first part of this chapter. Direct discrimination in the labour market and demographic and epidemiological changes in contemporary Chinese society are likely to produce increasing differentiation in the entitlements of women and men with consequences for their health and access to health care.

First, where women are discriminated against in recruitment and retention they are likely to suffer from breaks in their employment history which will reduce their employment-based entitlements and their ability to accumulate savings. Thus the elderly non-employed who lack viable income are currently vulnerable to low access to health care. Those previously employed by loss-making enterprises (both retired and laid off) or whose entitlements have become depleted face increasing financial difficulty and reliance on the support of their children. The greater tendency for older women to be in the laid-off category, combined with their slightly higher longevity, suggests an emerging greater vulnerability among this group. Elderly women are currently more likely than elderly men to have no source of pension or health insurance due to a lack of employment history. Laid-off workers, or those susceptible to being laid off, and casual workers may experience a loss of formal entitlements to women's health care services such as preventive screening and maternity services, as well as less access to all services as they age if they are unable to accumulate sufficient entitlements and assets.

Second, women are likely to face increasing pressures from societal or family expectations that they will take on the majority of the care burden associated with a demographic shift to an ageing population and an epidemiological transition to non-communicable diseases which are often chronic and therefore associated with a heavy care burden (an increasing ratio of elderly dependants with chronic diseases to younger workers and carers).[12] The emphasis on the 'quality' of the population that has accompanied the one-child policy is also creating increasing pressure on parents, and particularly women, to invest heavily in their child's upbringing, which involves significant time as well as financial inputs. In a climate of bias against women in employment this may encourage increased polarization in gender divisions of labour and roles, with an exaggeration of men's breadwinning role and women's caring role.

Our study found that in the case of severe illness, a heavy burden of care for the sick individual was placed on family members, and this burden fell particularly on women in the family. In several cases, elderly patients were also cared for by their children when they were ill. This applies both to care within health facilities and at home. In focus groups workers said that where nurse to patient ratios are low in hospital wards, they can only afford to employ carers if they have a relatively high salary. Even relatively elderly women can find themselves bearing heavy care burdens. A 76-year-old man who suffered from cerebral thrombosis was being cared for principally by his wife (of a similar age) and a woman in her sixties was caring for her daughter-in-law who had suffered a spinal haemorrhage. In one case already mentioned, a woman of 80, who suffered from chronic ill health herself, continued to care full time for her husband.

Women in the Nantong focus group also spoke of the pressure on them from their work and their household responsibilities:

> Now the pressure on women workers is great... the work is quite hard, but if you don't do it, jobs are hard to find... Towards the family, one's own life and feelings, the pressure is great... we have housework and looking after children. It's not like men. It's a heavy burden.

All these factors are likely to create an increasing number of 'dependants' (i.e. people who are not engaged in paid work due to other commitments in the long term or short term) who are disproportionately female. In the current benefits structure these individuals are unlikely to have direct entitlements and will also have less opportunity to accumulate savings. They are therefore likely to be reliant on others, with a negative impact on their independence and possibly on their health care seeking behaviour. The issue of how to ensure that carers and dependants (whether women or men) are adequately protected from loss of entitlements to health care is a crucial one for policy-makers to address.

In most cases women do not appear to be disadvantaged in the allocation of resources for health care in the household. However, some commentators argue that decision-making in many households is shifting towards men where their earning capacity advantage over women is increasing (Das Gupta *et al.*, 2000). This may lead to a decrease in women's confidence in their value in the household and a consequent self-imposed rationing of health care resources, as exemplified by the case studies of elderly female dependants.

Implications for Health Sector and Social Security Reform

The trends traced above have implications for health and social security reform. Current reforms are generally based on universal principles, which are not likely to take into account the gendered nature of the labour market and the different trajectories of women's employment. The allocation of formal entitlements to health care at the individual level appears to have benefited women historically by supporting their individual moral entitlements to care. However, as the socio-economic situation changes this may leave some women vulnerable to a loss of entitlements. Here, we summarize the main ways in which gender potentially has an impact on entitlements and their significance for reform.

Labour Market Discrimination

We have argued that discrimination in the labour market against women (particularly although not exclusively against older women with lower educational levels) reduces their health insurance entitlements, either because schemes are unable to offer benefits to laid-off or early retired workers or because individuals on short-term or temporary contracts have reduced insurance entitlements. Pathways for building entitlements to health insurance are needed for workers with short-term and temporary contracts, as are ways to strengthen the entitlements of workers who are retired early. These considerations require that a gender perspective be taken in the design of social security reforms, necessitating recognition of the different constraints and trajectories in women's and men's employment. Special attention needs to be paid to ensuring formal entitlements to preventive and curative women's health care services, including maternity services, by women with temporary or short-term contracts, and those working for loss-making enterprises, perhaps by de-linking insurance coverage for these services from individual employers.

We suggested that wage differentials between women and men, which are largely related to labour market segmentation, may also affect women's ability to accumulate savings which can be used to access health care, and that women's lack of independent income may reduce their willingness to use household resources to seek care for themselves. This trend has wide-reaching implications for women's position in the household, which extend beyond their access to health care, and raise fundamental questions about how to support gender equity through education and employment policy in a market economy. The development of medium- and long-term strategies to promote equal opportunities in both education and employment is necessary.

The Informal Care Economy

Women may be increasingly more vulnerable to being placed in a financially dependent position within the household as a result of the intersection of economic, social, demographic and epidemiological transitions in urban China. There are early indications that financial dependence on other family members is likely to reduce women's sense of their moral entitlements to health care. Provisions will need to be made for health care entitlements for carers, including mothers temporarily outside the labour market, and carers of the elderly and chronically sick. Such entitlements will need to be accessible to these groups in their own right as individuals, rather than through those who support them financially, to reduce the potential problems of these groups feeling a loss of moral entitlement to care.

Dependency

The death of a sole or main breadwinner increases the risk of a critical loss of entitlements by individuals and households. There is a need to provide safety nets which are sensitive to both women's and men's needs. For example, women are particularly vulnerable to a sudden loss of entitlements through widowhood or divorce if they have a low entitlements base at an individual level. Entitlements for widows (and widowers) or divorcees should therefore be strengthened and clarified under any emerging system.

Conclusion

Economic, social and demographic transitions in urban China are influencing entitlements to health care of individuals and households in complex ways. There is some evidence to suggest that gender is an emerging factor affecting formal and informal entitlements to health care access. A gender analysis of current trends suggests that gender differences and inequalities are likely to widen. Social security and health sector reforms need to take into account the ways in which gender interacts with other factors, such as age, education and cohort, to reduce the capacity of individuals to accumulate entitlements and to develop strategies to address specific vulnerabilities.

In order to capture gender differences, longitudinal studies are needed of changes in the opportunities and constraints for women of different ages and cohorts in the labour market and in household organization and relations. The potential vulnerabilities identified in this chapter may only just be emerging. Vulnerabilities may also take unexpected forms. Monitoring of social, demographic and employment trends using indicators disaggregated by gender is therefore essential.

Notes

1   For example, the People's Republic of China Labour Law states that women and men have equal rights to employment and that enterprises may not reject female employees on the basis of their gender or raise the standards for recruitment for female employees (with the exception of positions designated as 'unsuitable' for women by the State, such as mining) (Chapter 2, Article 13). The People's Republic of China Women's Rights Protection Law states that male and female workers should be paid the same wages for the same work (Article 23), women should not be discriminated against in promotion (Article 24), and employers cannot make women redundant on the basis of marriage, pregnancy, maternity leave or breast-feeding (Article 26).
2   Some firms in the 1980s and early 1990s offered 'return home' policies for women in which they paid women a proportion of their salaries to return home (Druschel, 1999).
3   An All China Women's Federation (ACWF) study in Shenzhen found that 67 per cent of the unemployed were women, rising to 73 per cent of those unemployed for more than a year (ACWF Women's Research Centre).

4 A fact-finding mission of the National People's Congress found in 1995 that employers were discriminating against female college graduates by setting age limits and higher requirements for female applicants, contrary to the law.

5 A study of rural migrants in Guangdong Province found that women were concentrated in the low paid jobs earning up to CNY500 per month, while men tended to have higher paid jobs, earning CNY500–800 (China Rights Forum, 1998).

6 For example, if a woman has worked for 35 years her pension will be 88 per cent of her salary, whilst if she has only worked for 20–30 years, her pension will be 75 per cent of her salary (China Rights Forum, 1998).

7 The ACWF found that the average income of laid-off men was CNY423 a month, whilst the average for women was CNY255, which was a greater income disparity than that amongst the waged.

8 This framework was first developed by Standing (2001).

9 The confidence interval (CI) indicates the range of values within which the true value of the parameter of interest is likely to lie in repeated samples.

10 Analysis of the National Health Service Survey (NHSS) data cited was carried out by Jun Gao, Centre for Health Statistics and Information, Ministry of Health, China in collaboration with Rachel Tolhurst and Shenglan Tang (Gao *et al.*, 2001).

11 The reason for this is that the data for the various 'vulnerable groups' has been aggregated because the small numbers for each group do not enable meaningful comparison between women and men.

12 In a situation where the available pool of jobs is decreasing this may also lead to a public pressure for women to 'return home' as has happened during the history of the People's Republic (Druschel, 1999).

Chapter 9

The Public Hospitals: Policy Reform, Productivity and Cost

Qingyue Meng, Clas Rehnberg, Ning Zhuang, Ying Bian and
Shenglan Tang

The hospital sector dominates the health care system in urban areas and consumes around 65 per cent of the total health expenditure. There was a rapid increase of 25 per cent per annum in hospital expenditures from the mid-1980s to mid-1990s (Ministry of Health, 1995). Influenced by national economic reforms, financial policies and administrative mechanisms for public hospitals have substantially changed since the early 1980s. In response to these changes, public hospitals adjusted their strategies in both administration and provision of health services. Both external and internal changes in the hospital sector are important to determine efficiency in the use of health resources and quality of services provided. The purpose of this chapter is to present the overall changes in hospital policies, hospital internal administration, productivity and cost in Zibo and Nantong. It starts by summarizing reforms surrounding public hospitals, and goes on to describe changes in administrative mechanisms taken by hospitals, analyse changes in productivity, quality and case mix and present out-patient and in-patient costs. The final sections discuss policy implications.

Hospital Sector Reform

The hospital sector reforms initiated in Zibo and Nantong followed the reform guidelines developed by central and provincial governments. Hence, the reform packages in both cities were quite similar. The reforms commenced in tandem with economic reform initiated in 1980. The main reform packages covered financial policy for public hospitals, health care pricing policy, health insurance system reform, regional health planning and community health care development.

Hospital Reimbursement Mechanism

Like other health authorities, the Zibo and Nantong local governments began to reform hospital reimbursement methods in the early 1980s. The major features of the reform were: user fees became an increasingly important source of revenue;

hospitals could retain all the surplus revenues for their own development; and hospitals were to have more financial autonomy (State Council, 1996). In the past two decades, the share of government budgets in total hospital revenue has rapidly decreased and user charges have become the major sources of hospital revenue. The reform of hospital reimbursement mechanisms in the two cities followed similar patterns, as summarized below.

- From 1950 to 1960, all revenues generated by public hospitals were handed over to treasury authorities and recurrent expenses of hospitals were totally covered by government subsidies. Hospital accounting was very complex and difficult to manage.
- From 1960 to 1979, public hospitals were subsidized by government funding to cover the salaries of health workers. Incomes from user fees were retained by hospitals to cover other recurrent costs. In 1965, 90 per cent of spending on health workers' salaries was subsidized by government funding. In 1979, financial resources from government budgets in public hospitals stood at 135 per cent of health workers' salaries. During this period, prices were set far below recurrent costs. Government funding was the major source of finance.
- From 1979 to the present, the allocation of government subsidies was based on the number of hospital beds or a defined volume of medical services. Prices of medical services began to be adjusted. The share of government funding in total hospital revenue decreased rapidly. User fees and drug mark-ups became the major source of finance. At present, about 30 per cent of salary costs is funded by government and about 5 per cent of hospital revenues comes from government. The economic autonomy of hospitals has increased: all revenues generated by hospitals are retained and used by the hospitals themselves.

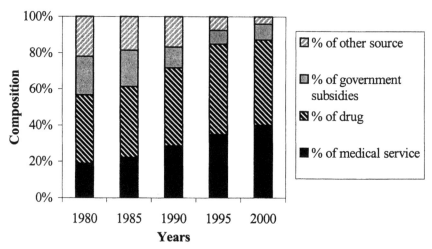

Figure 9.1 Hospital incomes composition in selected years in China
Source: Ministry of Health (2001).

Figure 9.1 presents hospital incomes and their sources in selected years between 1980 and 2000 for public hospitals for the country. User charges for medical services and drugs increased during the two decades. Revenues generated from the provision of medical services and drugs come from out-of-pocket payments or third party payers. The latter mainly includes GIS and LIS. The government subsidies in the figure do not include subsidies allocated to the government health insurance scheme.

Pricing Policies

The reform of the health care pricing policy was initiated by the central government from 1980 after a long-term implementation of a 'low price' policy. The initial purpose of this reform was to compensate public hospitals for the fall in the relative contribution of government budgets. Since then, a new health care pricing system has been established. In this system, responsibilities of various government agencies in setting and regulating prices are defined, methods of setting and adjusting prices are developed, and the use of an official fee schedule for hospital to charge health care users is regulated. The State Development Planning Commission is responsible for defining the principles for setting health care prices, in collaboration with the Ministries of Health and Finance. Provincial or municipal government agencies, led by the Department of Price Administration, develop and adjust concrete fee schedules for implementation in public hospitals. The fee items in the official schedules are procedures of medical services. There were large variations in the number of fee items across provinces, ranging from 2,500 to 5,000, in the year 2000. The stated method of pricing those items is cost-based, implying that fee rate should reflect cost level for each fee item.

The official regulations require health facilities to adhere to the fee schedule issued by their provincial or prefecture governments. Provincial and municipal Departments of Price Administration and Health organize regulatory activities examining and monitoring the compliance of hospitals with the official fee schedule. Hospitals are fined for overcharging patients. Public hospitals at and above county level are required to set up price self-regulation mechanisms. Part- or full-time hospital staff in each hospital should be employed to monitor the implementation of official schedules in clinical departments within the hospital. In recent years, the central and local governments also request hospitals to post the major official fee rates in hospital public places to the patients.

In Shandong and Jiangsu Provinces about 4,000 fee items were used before 2000 (Shandong Provincial Government, 2000; Jiangsu Provincial Government, 1999). In 1980, the Shandong Provincial Government set the first version of the fee schedule to be used in all public hospitals. In 1989 and 1990, a decade after the publication of the first fee schedule, the prices of some diagnostic and surgical services were raised. In 1992 and 1993, prices of some diagnostic services using high-tech medical equipment were reduced, while prices of some labour-intensive medical services were raised. In 1994, the second version of the fee schedule was set. The fee schedule currently used in Shandong Province is the 2000 version.

Jiangsu Province had a similar process with regard to adjusting the fee schedules of hospital services. Before 1993, prices of high-tech diagnostic and treatment service items were set much higher than their costs, compared with basic health services. In 1993, the fee schedule was adjusted by reducing the prices of high-tech services such as CT scans and magnetic resonance imaging (MRI), and increasing the prices of registration fees and bed fees. All patients, regardless of their health insurance status, were charged the same prices. In 1997, in accordance with urban health insurance reform, prices of medical professional services and non-essential services were increased and prices of CT and MRI reduced. In addition, price regulation was strengthened.

Health Insurance Reform

The Chinese government has launched reforms of urban health insurance with the aim of the eventual establishment of a universal and affordable health care system in cities. Different pilot studies for the reform were carried out in the mid-1990s and generalized in late 2000. The evolution from the original GIS and LIS systems in Zibo and Nantong has been described in Chapter 4. Urban health insurance reform in China included cost-containment measures on both the demand and supply sides. While co-payments were established for the insured, measures such as the adoption of alternative payment methods and increased use of contracting of providers were taken for health service suppliers.

Nantong commenced radical reform of urban health insurance from April 1997, as one of 57 national pilot cities. At the outset the municipal government took a series of political and administrative measures. Policy documents, including 'Design of the Employee-Based Health Insurance Scheme', 'Methods of Managing the Health Insurance Fund', 'Methods of Contracting Hospitals for the Urban Health Insurance Scheme', and 'Regulation of Health Insurance Fund Collection Procedures', were issued and the policies implemented. In addition, a specific organization, the Nantong Health Insurance Management Centre, was established within the Municipal Labour and Social Security Bureau. The major differences in the system between Nantong and Zibo were that changes in payment methods, pooling of the insurance fund and selection of contract hospitals were not found in Zibo during the study period.

Regional Health Planning and the Community Health System

There are several approaches for controlling and monitoring the community health system. In 1992, Zibo's Zhoucun district was involved in an experiment to reform the methods of health resource distribution and allocation. The purpose of the reform was to increase efficiency and equity by adjusting the existing pattern of resource allocation. According to the reform package, local government has the authority to plan the distribution of Zibo's available health resources regardless of the ownership of the resources. By doing this, it was hoped that duplication of facilities and functions would be avoided and more resources could be transferred from high-level hospitals to community health centres. This reform did not achieve its expected outcome owing to the complex political and administrative procedures involved in managing health resources.

Since 1980, the community health care system in urban cities has been largely destroyed. An increase in hospital autonomy and the cancellation of the referral system are the major reasons. An incomplete system of health service delivery at the community level explained in part the rapid increase in medical costs. One of the strategies being employed in Zibo to control the unreasonable escalation of medical costs is the re-establishment of the community health care system. Community health centres and stations to provide curative and preventive services have been established. Some health workers previously working in hospitals are now working in these centres. The success of this reform will benefit both regional health resource planning and health insurance reform, because the redistribution of health resources will increase system efficiency. However, this reform will take a long time and should gradually receive stronger political support.

Hospital Management and Administration

Characteristics of Sample Hospitals

Table 9.1 Characteristics of sample hospitals in Zibo and Nantong

Indicators	1990	1995	1997	1999
Zibo				
Number of health workers	5,110	6,320	6,800	7,020
Number of hospital beds	4,030	4,820	5,400	5,500
Total revenues (CNY10,000)	830	1,400	2,000	2,700
% of government share	11	6	6	5
% of user fee	35	40	38	41
% of drugs	48	46	47	46
Total value of high-tech equipment (CNY million)	23	44	76	120
Nantong				
Number of health worker	5,501	6,657	7,011	7,340
Number of hospital beds	4,553	5,289	5,750	5,950
Total revenues (CNY10,000)	1,400	2,500	3,300	4,300
% of government share	7	6	5	6
% of user fee	32	35	36	39
% of drugs	53	49	49	50
Total value of high-tech equipment (CNY million)	17	64	92	130

The analysis of the efficiency in production in the two cities was based on a sample of county-level hospitals. In Zibo and Nantong all the hospitals sampled were at and above county (district) level. Of the 22 hospitals in Zibo, 2 hospitals were at municipal level and the rest were at county level. In the sample, 11 were general hospitals, 8 were Chinese traditional hospitals and 3 hospitals were owned by enterprises. In Nantong, of the 19 hospitals, 10 were general hospitals, 8 were Chinese traditional hospitals and 1 was an enterprise hospital. The characteristics of sample hospitals are presented in Table 9.1.

Changes in Scales of Hospitals

The change of investment in capital and high-tech equipment is substantially higher than that for labour and beds for both cities. Regarding revenues, the development reflects the increase of revenues from drugs and user fees. Government revenues have become less important for the hospital sector.

Changes in hospital scales in Zibo can be summarized as follows:

- From 1990 to 1995, the annual increase rates of health workers was 4 per cent, hospital beds 3.7 per cent and value of high-tech equipment 14 per cent. With regard to total revenues, shares of government budgets decreased from 11 per cent to 6 per cent, user fees increased from 35 per cent to 40 per cent, and revenues from drugs decreased from 48 per cent to 46 per cent.
- From 1995 to 1997, the annual increase rates of health workers was 3.2 per cent, hospital beds 5.8 per cent and value of high-tech equipment 32 per cent. Regarding total revenues, shares of government budget remained at 6 per cent and user fees slightly decreased.
- From 1997 to 1999, the annual increase rates of health workers was 1.2 per cent, hospital beds 1 per cent and value of high-tech equipment 25 per cent. Regarding total revenues, shares of government budget decreased from 6 per cent to 5 per cent and user fees increased from 38 per cent to 41 per cent.

Changes in hospital scales in Nantong can be summarized as follows:

- From 1990 to 1995, the annual increase rates of health workers was 4.4 per cent, hospital beds 3.0 per cent and value of high-tech equipment 30.6 per cent. Regarding total revenues, shares of government budget decreased from 7 per cent to 6 per cent, user fees increased from 32 per cent to 35 per cent, and revenues from drugs decreased from 53 per cent to 49 per cent.
- From 1995 to 1997, the annual increase rates of health workers was 2.6 per cent, hospital beds 4.3 per cent and value of high-tech equipment 19.6 per cent. Regarding total revenues, shares of government budget reduced by 1 per cent and user fees slightly increased.
- From 1997 to 1999, the annual increase rates of health workers was 2.3 per cent, hospital beds 1.7 per cent and value of high-tech equipment 17.1 per cent. Regarding total revenues, shares of government budget slightly increased and user fees increased from 36 per cent to 39 per cent.

The major difference in changes in hospital scales between Zibo and Nantong was that, after 1997, the increase rate of the value of high-tech equipment was slower in Nantong than in Zibo.

Responsibility System

In order to improve the performance of clinical departments and individual health workers, a responsibility system was introduced in the hospital sector in Nantong in 1993 and in Zibo in 1994. This system is an internally administrated mechanism designed and implemented by the hospitals themselves. At the beginning of a year, the hospital leadership and department heads negotiate a contract in which responsibilities and incentives are defined. There are some differences between the systems in Zibo and Nantong. However, there are usually four key components in the contract: volume of workloads, quality, incomes and patient satisfaction:

- Workloads: out-patient encounters and in-patient days are the measures of workloads. The determination of volumes of workloads that each clinical department should provide are based on the workloads delivered in the last year.
- Quality: about 50 indicators are designed to assess service quality. These indicators cover quality, structure, process and outcome. Scoring out of 100 for each indicator is used.
- Income: methods for calculating the incomes of departments vary across hospitals. The basic formula is: Incomes = Revenues – Expenditures.
- Patient satisfaction: the number of incidents of misconduct in practice is the key indicator.

Indicators and scoring methods are generalized in an evaluation manual. A specific department within hospitals is responsible for conducting a monthly assessment according to the scoring manual. The sum of the scores each department gains is the basis upon which hospital managers allocate bonuses. Within departments, the heads will distribute bonuses to individual workers according to their performances. However, there is no scoring system within the department.

This system has, to some extent, improved the performance of departments within hospitals and encouraged health workers to increase their productivity. However, the gap in income levels among doctors and nurses working in different hospital departments has increased significantly. Health workers who attended the focus group discussions reported that part of the gap is seen as reasonable, since people's workloads and skills differ. Nonetheless, some of the income gap was attributed purely to the differences in medical equipment used by different departments. Prices for the use of different medical equipment vary a great deal. In other words, the marginal profits from the use of different equipment were not the same. One doctor said in a focus group discussion that the machines were making money for hospitals and providing bonuses for health workers. This implies that it is not easy to establish a good system that provides fair and acceptable incentives to health workers and that ensures rational provision of quality services.

Personnel Policy

Hospital directors are appointed by the same level of government. Directors of hospitals decide who fill the roles of department heads. From 1996, personnel policy started to be reformed in Zibo and Nantong, in accordance with guidelines issued by central government. The permanent relationship between health workers and hospitals was changed into a contractual relationship. The new policy allows hospital management to fire and hire staff. First, positions required by hospitals are defined according to service patterns and workloads. Second, a competition mechanism is used to select health workers to work in the defined positions. Finally, health workers who are not successful in the competition will lose their jobs or will be transferred to non-professional positions. However, in practice, this policy has not been well implemented for many reasons. Key informant interviews with hospital managers in the two cities reflected that hospitals could not refuse applicants if those people were recommended by senior officials, and that hospital managers were not able to fire employees if no new positions for the fired staff were found within the hospitals.

Pricing Practice

The fee schedule in the hospital sector is assumed to follow the stipulated fee schedule. However, no hospital in Zibo and Nantong charged patients strictly according to the fee schedule issued from the Shandong and Jiangsu provincial governments. The topic of actual prices charged to the patients was too sensitive to obtain answers from hospital managers in either Zibo or Nantong. In Zibo we were able to investigate this matter by examining information on two areas: (1) the number of hospitals that were punished because of illegal behaviour in charging users. From discussions with health officials who were responsible for regulating prices, it was found that in 1990 five hospitals were punished by the price administration agency. In 1997 and 1999, six and seven hospitals were punished; and (2) differences in fee levels between official prices and prices in practice. An investigation conducted in Shandong showed that in 15 hospitals, including three hospitals in Zibo, the prices were double official prices.

Health officials interviewed in this study attributed this situation to the delay in fee schedule adjustment. Because fee schedules had not been updated at the same time as the changes in prices of health inputs, hospitals found it very hard to implement schedules if they wanted to maintain a financial balance. Key informants indicated that, in most cases, hospitals could not cover operating costs with government budgets and revenues generated from user charges with the standard fee schedules. Usually, the hospitals distorted standard fee schedules through: separating one fee item into two or more fee items (hospitals generate additional revenues from charging patients for the 'new' service items); providing more profitable services and fewer non-profitable services (for example, high-tech equipment services and drugs may be oversupplied); and introducing new service items. For service items that were not included in the fee schedules, the hospital could apply for new prices if those services were to be carried out by the hospital.

In most cases, the prices of those new service items would be set at a high level, which stimulates hospitals to introduce new service items.

Bonus System

In order to stimulate the health workers to increase their productivity, the bonus system was introduced in the hospital sector in Nantong in 1985 and in Zibo in 1987. There are four time periods for different types of bonus system. In Zibo, from 1987 to 1990 a flat bonus method was operated. With this method, every health worker was awarded the same bonus regardless of his or her contribution. From 1990 to 1994, two methods of distributing bonuses were adopted in the studied hospitals. One was a volume-based method and the other was an income-based method. The former means that rewards were distributed to a health worker or a department according to the volume of services (out-patient visits and in-patient days) the health worker or department provided. The latter was based on the revenues a health worker or a department generated by providing medical services. Since 1994, a performance-based bonus method has been used. Elements of performance include revenues generated, quality of services and volume of services. Revenues are still central in this method. Nantong experienced the same changes in implementing different bonus methods as Zibo.

Because the bonus systems used in the two cities were based on volume of services and amount of revenues, the departments of hospitals would try to generate more revenues through providing more services. This could be one of the reasons for the cost escalation of medical care. In addition, the overuse of diagnostic tests was also reported by some service users participating in the focus group discussions in both of the study cities. Some service users clearly understood that some doctors wanted their patients to take as many tests as possible, even if some of the tests were not necessary for making a correct diagnosis. They knew that some hospitals would like to generate revenues by providing more services to their patients.

Performance

Different indicators could be used for assessing the performance of the hospital sector. The hospital records and the official statistics allow us to estimate labour-productivity measures and throughputs such as: out-patient services per doctor, bed-days per doctor, income per health worker, bed occupancy rate, length of stay (LOS) and bed turnover rate. Out-patient service has been adjusted with quality, price and case mix. Bed-days have been adjusted with quality and price. Income has been adjusted with price. The results are summarized in Table 9.2.

In Zibo both out-patient visits and in-patient days served by each doctor decreased from 1990 to 1999, especially bed-days per doctor. The volume of in-patient services reduced by about 200 bed-days per doctor from 1990 to 1999. Bed occupancy rates also decreased from 81 per cent in 1990 to 63 per cent in 1999. In the same period, income generated by each health worker increased rapidly, from

CNY17,000 in 1990 to CNY46,000 in 1999. A similar pattern is shown for Nantong. Out-patient visits and in-patient days served by each doctor decreased from 1990 to 1999. Between 1990 and 1999 out-patient visits per doctor reduced by 27 per cent and bed-days per doctor reduced by 36 per cent. In the same period, the income generated by each health worker increased rapidly, from CNY16,070 in 1990 to CNY66,270 in 1999.

Table 9.2 Hospital performance in Zibo and Nantong in selected years

	1990	1995	1997	1999
Zibo				
Out-patient and emergency visits per doctor	1,312	1,166	1,217	1,218
Bed-days per doctor	690	574	525	486
LOS (days)	17.4	15.6	14.2	12.4
Income per health worker (CNY)	17,033	27,150	34,631	46,011
Bed turnover rate (times)	19	19	19	21
Bed occupancy rate (%)	81	73	66	63
Nantong				
Out-patient and emergency visits per doctor	1,928	1,150	1,101	1,099
Bed-days per doctor	806	561	532	513
LOS (days)	20.2	17.3	15.9	15.0
Income per health worker (CNY)	19,270	55,443	72,576	84,214
Bed turnover rate (times)	19	16	16	17
Bed occupancy rate (%)	95	71	64	64

To sum up, hospitals seem to do less but increase their financial performance. The development is to some extent similar to an international trend with a shift from in-patient care to out-patient care. However, the decline in out-patient care is difficult to explain. There are other factors affecting the decline in productivity in the study hospitals of the two cities. First, the use of out-patient and in-patient services during the 1990s has declined for several reasons, including the rapid increase of medical care costs, the reduced coverage of work-related health insurance and rising competition in the medical care market. In-depth interviews with hospital managers in the two cities highlighted this problem. Second, as reported by the hospital managers, it is very difficult for the hospitals to lay off health workers and staff, even if they do not have much work to do, although in theory they have the right to hire and fire staff. In addition, these hospitals sometimes had to take on military officers who just retired from the service and new medical graduates, according to government rules.

Figures 9.2 and 9.3 shows changes in hospital productivity by hospital type in the two cities. The development in Zibo shows a similar pattern for all types of hospital apart from the enterprise hospitals where out-patient care per doctor has increased. The development in Nantong is very similar across the hospitals. Overall the development in the two cities shows a similar pattern.

Table 9.3 presents the unit costs of health services by type of hospital in both cities without adjustments of health care quality and case mix.

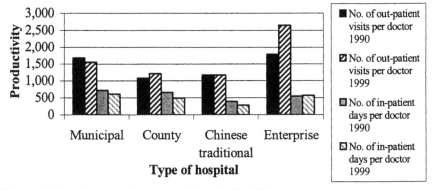

Figure 9.2 Productivity by type of hospital in Zibo

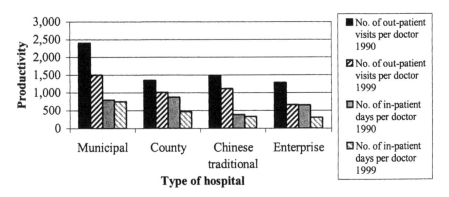

Figure 9.3 Productivity by type of hospital in Nantong

Table 9.3 Unit costs by type of hospital in Zibo and Nantong (without adjustments of quality and case mix)

	Municipal general hospital		County general hospital		Chinese traditional hospital		Enterprise hospital	
	Zibo	Nantong	Zibo	Nantong	Zibo	Nantong	Zibo	Nantong
Unit cost of out-patient visit								
1990	32.9	20.5	51.7	22.2	11.5	16.8	16.1	47.8
1995	54.8	59.7	38.6	58.1	31.7	58.5	34.4	74.9
1997	67.3	76.9	52.1	75.4	37.4	76.6	55.8	91.3
1999	104.7	82.9	63.3	91.0	52.1	100.2	74.3	116.5
Unit cost of bed-day								
1990	83.8	109.2	72.2	68.7	89.2	64.9	26.5	67.2
1995	178.5	203.1	107.4	168.1	212.1	300.9	81.4	151.2
1997	220.4	272.6	157.2	220.0	286.4	353.9	144.1	207.9
1999	223.2	314.9	218.9	275.3	399.6	382.8	243.3	166.5

Quality and Case Mix of Hospital Services

The figures presented above could be considered as labour productivity measures and throughputs of hospital services. A problem with these indicators is that the cost of inputs, such as labour, drugs and capital, is not considered. Another problem is the change of quality over time and across units. In order to compare the unit cost of hospital services, quality and case mix in different time periods and among hospitals were adjusted.

Adjustment of Quality

Comparison of unit cost of different hospitals requires that quality of care should be adjusted to be equal across the hospitals. In this study, a quality adjusted index (QAI) was used to adjust the quality of sample hospitals. The formula for calculating QAI is:

$$QAI = X = \sum_{i=1}^{n} X_i / S_i * W_i \qquad (1)$$

Where X_i are the factual numbers of indicators, S_i are the standard numbers of indicators, and W_i are the weights representing importance of selected indicators in determining quality. X_i were obtained from the survey, S_i were set by the Ministry of Health, and W_i were provided by medical experts. From 50 indicators that are usually used for assessing the quality of hospital services, six were selected by a panel of medical experts. Selected indicators include recovery rates of hospitalized patients, consistent rates of diagnosis before and after discharge of in-patients, consistent rates of diagnosis before and after physical operations, rates of successfully rescuing emergency cases, rates of qualified nursing and hospital infectious rates. Those indicators represent key procedures of diagnosis, treatment, and nursing in out-patient, in-patient and surgical care facilities. Table 9.4 shows the variables for measuring QAI.

Table 9.4 Indicators used for calculating the quality adjusted index

Indicators	S_i(%)	Weights
Recovery rates of hospitalized patients	≥93.7	0.190
Consistent rates of diagnosis before and after discharges	≥95.0	0.172
Consistent rates of diagnosis before and after physical operations	≥90.0	0.170
Rates of successfully rescuing emergency cases	≥80.0	0.185
Rates of qualified nursing work	≥90.0	0.172
Hospital internal infectious rates	≤10.0	0.126

The above figures for each hospital were substituted into formula (1). Values of QAI of each hospital in 1999 were obtained as listed above. There are no considerable variations in values of QAI among the hospitals. Values of QAI in 1990, 1995, and 1997 were also calculated. Those values are used in the productivity calculation.

In Figure 9.4 the development of the quality of services delivered in the two city hospitals is presented. The indicator is based on the methodology described above and shows a positive trend. The values of quality index were 1.05 in 1990 and 1.07 in 1999 in Zibo. In Nantong, the values of quality index were 1.03 in 1990 and 1.08 in 1999. Improvement of quality between 1990 and 1999 was greater in Nantong than in Zibo.

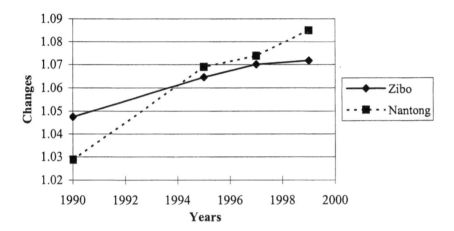

Figure 9.4 Changes in service quality

The values of the quality index were slightly different between different levels of hospital. In Zibo the value of quality index was 1.08 in municipal hospitals, while it was 1.06 in county (district) hospitals. In Nantong values of quality index in municipal and county (district) hospitals were 1.09 and 1.07 respectively.

Adjustment of Case Mix

Apart from taking the changes in quality into consideration, it is also important to estimate the effect of changes in case mix in order to analyse hospitals' productivity. The severity of illness has close relation with medical expenses. Patients with severe conditions cost more than others. The adjustment of case mix for in-patient services was based on the diagnosis. A case mix index (CMI) that is widely used for such adjustment was employed. The formula to calculate CMI is as follows.

$$CMI_j = \sum(C_j X^* P_j X)/\sum(CX^* PX) \qquad (2)$$

Where CMI_j is the value of CMI of j hospital, C_jX is the average expense of j hospital, CX is the standard expense of X disease, P_j is the proportion of patients with X disease in j hospital, and PX is the proportion of patients with X diseases in total patients of sample hospitals. By considering the differences in the share of patients with different diseases the total output could be weighted. For out-patient services there is a lack of diagnosis data. In the study, the average expense per out-patient service was used to adjust the case mix of out-patient services. In order to avoid unstable expenses across years, the medical expenses of each hospital in the four selected years were averaged (Table 9.5).

Table 9.5 Results of case mix adjustment

Hospital level	Values of CMI
Zibo	
Out-patient services municipal hospitals	0.98
Out-patient services county hospitals	0.78
In-patient services municipal hospitals	1.33
In-patient services county hospitals	0.98
Nantong	
Out-patient services municipal hospitals	1.11
Out-patient services county hospitals	0.98
In-patient services municipal hospitals	1.67
In-patient services county hospitals	0.84

The calculation of the case mix index showed difference in its values between different levels of hospitals in Zibo and Nantong. Values of the case mix index in municipal hospitals were greater than those in county (district) hospitals.

Unit Costs for Hospital Services

The unit cost for both in-patient and out-patient services was calculated for Zibo and Nantong. All costs and expenditures have been converted to fixed prices using 1999 as a base year. In both cities, unit costs per out-patient visit and per bed-day increased rapidly from 1990 to 1999. The growth rate of unit cost per bed-day was greater than the unit cost per out-patient visit (Figure 9.5).

In Zibo the unit cost per out-patient visit was 2.75 times higher in 1999 than that in 1990. The annual increase rates of unit cost per out-patient visit was 11 per cent from 1990 to 1995, 14 per cent from 1995 to 1997, and 13 per cent from 1997 to 1999. From 1995 to 1999 the unit cost per bed-day increased nearly four times. Annual increase rates per bed-day were 14 per cent from 1990 to 1995, 18 per cent from 1995 to 1999, and nearly 20 per cent from 1997 to 1999.

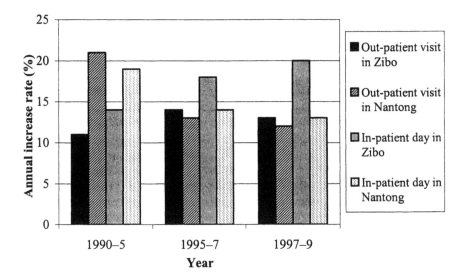

Figure 9.5 Unit cost in Zibo and Nantong in selected years

In Nantong the unit cost per out-patient visit was 4.08 times higher in 1999 than that in 1990, an annual increase rate of 17 per cent. Annual increase rates of the unit cost per out-patient visit was 21 per cent from 1990 to 1995, 13 per cent from 1995 to 1997, and 12 per cent from 1997 to 1999. From 1995 to 1999 the unit cost per bed-day increased nearly four times. Annual increase rates per bed-day were 19 per cent from 1990 to 1995, 14 per cent from 1995 to 1999, and 13 per cent from 1997 to 1999. It is also obvious that the overall level of unit costs in Nantong is higher than that in Zibo. However, from 1997 the increase rates of unit costs were less in Nantong than in Zibo.

The development of the unit cost also differs across the types of hospital. Figures 9.6 and 9.7 present the unit costs of different types of hospital in the two cities. In Zibo the unit costs of both out-patient and in-patient services in enterprise hospitals increased more rapidly than those in other types of hospital. From 1990 to 1999, the unit cost per out-patient visit increased by 4.5 times and the unit cost per bed day increased by 9.1 times in enterprise hospitals. County (district) general hospitals had the lowest increase rates, whereas in Nantong the unit costs in enterprise hospitals had the lowest increase rate.

The main reason why the unit costs increased significantly in the 1990s, and particularly in the early 1990s, might be related to the fact that, while the use of services declined in the two cities as a whole, the revenues generated by the vast majority of hospitals surveyed increased over the period. Induced demand for expensive diagnostic tests and treatment may be partly attributed to the increase of unit costs. In addition, the improvement in quality of the services provided by these hospitals, as presented above, might also consume more health resources.

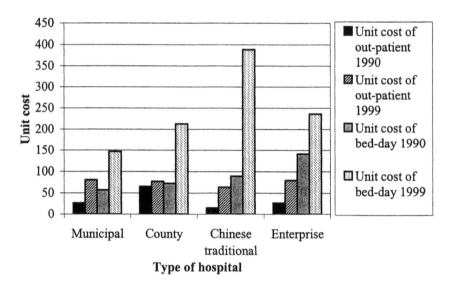

Figure 9.6 Unit cost by type of hospital in Zibo

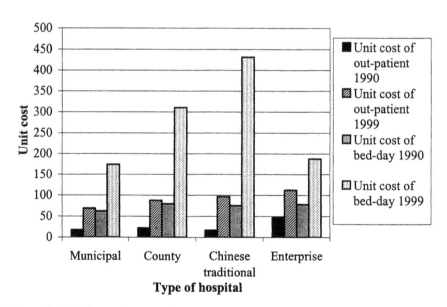

Figure 9.7 Unit cost by type of hospital in Nantong

Discussion

The stated aims of health sector reform were to improve the efficiency of service provision, to contain the escalation of medical costs, to improve access to health care and to improve service quality. Since about three-quarters of health resources were allocated to the hospital sector, the performance of hospitals would determine whether or not those aims could be achieved. The top priority of hospitals is to maintain a financial balance. This is also the precondition for hospitals to remain in operation. Therefore, any actions of hospitals in response to changes in their environment, including financial polices, would ultimately be directed towards the realization of financial viability.

Since the early 1980s, hospital financial reform has been central to all reform strategies in the health sector. When the government decided to allow the market to play a more important role in the financing of hospital services, it marked the beginning of hospitals having to generate revenues largely from user fees and drug mark-ups. Due to the fact that the mechanisms of the planned economy had dominated hospital procedures for a long time, in attempting to generate surplus revenue hospital administrators and managers lacked the knowledge and skills to plan cost-effective, efficient organizational strategies.

When the government budget was allocated according to the numbers of hospital staff and beds, hospitals simply recruited more health workers and equipped more hospital beds. When the government set high prices for high-tech services, hospitals purchased more high-technology equipment. When the government could not adjust the fee schedules in line with inflation, hospitals distorted the prices of medical services. When the government fixed the mark-up rates for drugs, hospitals planned to use new and expensive drugs. The rationale for other hospital actions, such as the implementations of the bonus and responsibility systems, also revolved around the primary objective of hospitals, that of maintaining a financial balance. Because the hospital sector was not effectively regulated and the financial responsibility of government was not clearly defined, it was hard to monitor and regulate the hospital actions mentioned above. In recent years it has been generally agreed that hospital financial reform is the root cause of changes in the hospital sector (Zhao, 1998; Liu, 1991).

It is hoped that urban health insurance reform, by changing the payment system and contractual relationship, could have positive effects on the efficiency of hospital resource usage (Zheng, 1996; Cai, 1999; Yang, 1997). However, it should be noted that, in general, only a small proportion of health care users in hospitals are covered by health insurance schemes. Therefore, the relationship between urban health insurance reform and the efficient performance of hospitals is not clear at the macro level. Some recent changes in the insurance system will be examined in Chapter 10.

This study revealed that hospital productivity in both Zibo and Nantong has decreased over the past decade. Each doctor provided fewer out-patient and in-patient services and the bed occupancy rates decreased. The findings are consistent with results of other studies. Out-patient visits served by each health worker declined from 575 in 1992 to 504 in 1997, according to the National Health

Service Survey (Ministry of Health, 1999a). It was reported that the occupancy rates of hospital beds decreased from 85 per cent in 1994 to 69 per cent in 1997 (Ministry of Health, 2000). The number of out-patient visits and hospital bed-days provided by each doctor are determined by two factors: changes in the total quantities of out-patient visits and hospital bed-days; and changes in the number of doctors. If the increase in demand for hospital services is less than the increase in the number of doctors, out-patient visits and hospital bed-days per doctor would certainly decline.

In recent years, the demand for hospital services did not increase proportionally in line with increases in household incomes and population rates. In general, in the 1990s hospital care utilization decreased. The reasons identified include self-treatment and the financial hardship of the users, and the quality of health care (Luo and Hu, 1998; Du *et al.*, 1998). In Zibo and Nantong the annual increase rate of the demand for hospital services was less than the natural growth rate of the population in the 1990s. In the meantime, increases in hospital staff rates remained high, which resulted in a reduction in the productivity of hospital provision.

Three reasons could account for the rapid increase in the number of hospital staff. First, the expansion of the labour force in the hospital sector was mainly directed by government policy on medical student recruitment. The Chinese government has tried to address the problem of the shortage in health resources since 1980 through a number of measures. These include strengthening the capability of the formal medical education sector by training more students, permitting the private sector to run medical educational and training activities, and reintroducing private practice in the health sector. In 1986, 390,000 medical students graduated from 130 medical universities. In 1995, the number of medical educational institutions and graduated medical students had increased to 177 and 805,400, respectively (Ministry of Health and Ministry of Education, 2000). Second, government budgeting policy strongly encouraged public hospitals to recruit more health workers. Before 1998, government funding allocated to public hospitals was partially determined by the number of hospital workers: more health workers implied higher government subsidies. Third, public hospitals lacked autonomy in formulating personnel policy. At present in China, public hospitals have very limited autonomy over employing hospital staff, even though central government has called for adjustments to hospital staff recruitment in accordance with the changes in demand which commenced in 1996. Usually, public hospital managers cannot refuse applicants for hospital employment if those people are introduced by government authorities. Meanwhile, hospitals also experience difficulty in dismissing employees, even if they are surplus to requirements.

Recently, a new 'Doctor Law' has been implemented to control the number of doctors practising medicine. All doctors, except very elderly ones and new medical graduates, are now required to pass a qualifying examination before they are awarded a licence. However, one health administrator interviewed thought that the current examination was too easy to achieve its intended purpose. Therefore, the problem of overstaffing in many hospitals in the two cities was reported in several focus group discussions and in-depth interviews.

In Zibo and Nantong, unit costs per out-patient visit and bed-day increased rapidly from 1990 to 1999. In terms of the annual increase rate of unit costs, hospitals in Zibo and Nantong experienced different patterns. The annual increase rates of unit costs of hospitals in Zibo rose continuously during different periods. In Nantong, the annual increase rates of unit costs declined from 1995. A country-wide hospital survey revealed that unit costs underwent a similar increase in the 1990s (Meng *et al.*, 1998). In another study (Xu, 2001) about 30 per cent of costs were not necessary for the treatment of the diseases.

Because the calculations of unit costs have been adjusted with case mix and quality of health care in this study, possible explanations for the rapid rise in unit costs could include the following: the increase in prices of inputs, including staff salaries and medical materials and drugs; the use of high-technology equipment; and the oversupply of health workers, hospital beds and treatment.

Staff salaries and the prices of medical supplies are not controlled by hospitals. In addition, to a large extent the prices of drugs are determined by the pharmaceutical producers and distributors. The annual increase rates of salaries and medical supplies were 10.8 per cent and 7 per cent, respectively, between 1990 and 1999 (National Bureau of Statistics, 2000; Zibo Bureau of Statistics, 2001). The price factor could not fully explain the dramatic increase in the unit prices of hospital services. Other explanations such as over-prescription of drugs, overuse of high-tech equipment, and a surplus of hospital resources would be crucial in determining levels of unit costs.

Revenues generated from drugs have become one of the major sources of finance for hospital operations since the mid-1980s. In terms of unit cost, more than 50 per cent of expenses were allocated to drugs in the two cities. Specifically, the fixed mark-up rate of drugs induces hospitals to use more expensive drugs. Even though policy-makers and regulators paid great attention to the control of drug costs, the effects on cost containment were not satisfied during the study period. Findings from key informant interviews also confirmed that the close link between drug prescription and hospital revenues had distorted the drug prescription behaviour. A number of research reports document the fact that new and expensive drugs are usually the first choice by some doctors in hospitals (Li, 1998; Wang, 1999).

Overuse of high technologies certainly resulted in a rise in medical costs. Because hospitals could benefit from providing high-tech services in accordance with the pricing policy before 1995, all secondary and tertiary hospitals in Zibo and Nantong purchased CT scanners and other kinds of high-technology equipment. Use of these technologies increased the cost of medical services and, moreover, hospitals would try to use them as much as possible to generate revenue. As a result, incidences of unnecessary service provision using these technologies would increase. In 1995, prices of high-tech services were reduced in the two cities. However, by that time a great deal of high-tech equipment had been purchased by most of the hospitals. The escalation of unit costs in hospitals was also caused by the rapid expansion of other types of health resources, such as hospital staff. The explanations are similar to those provided in the hospital productivity analysis.

Recommendations

The success of the Chinese health care system before 1980 is closely associated with health financing policy. Strong intervention from government assured the accessibility and affordability of health care for most of the population. Rural cooperative medical systems and urban government and labour health insurance schemes were largely supported by the low-cost health care system. The referral system, primary health care development, investment in public health programmes, and the limitation of high-technology investment were the major determinants of low-level health care costs.

Economic reform initiated in the early 1980s basically changed the whole economic structure and people's lives. The introduction of the competitive mechanism is one of the key reform issues. Most goods and services produced are determined by market forces and no longer by the government. This new kind of mechanism greatly improved economic productivity and increased economic freedom. In a very short period of time, the Chinese economy progressed enormously.

Health care development has benefited from economic reform: more hospitals were constructed with the newly generated wealth; the health workforce was strengthened owing to the expansion of medical education; hospitals were equipped with better and higher technologies, absorbing a large proportion of investment in this area; and newer and more drugs were used in hospitals with the rapid increase of domestic and foreign pharmaceutical products. In addition, hospitals were encouraged to provide more services because of changes in the incentive structure and the introduction of a competitive market in the hospital sector.

However, market forces can produce negative effects in the health sector if the government cannot effectively regulate the imperfections in the market and merely intends to the use market mechanism to address all the problems in health care. Hospital financing reform, as a result of economic reform, has caused a series of problems in the health sector, including cost escalation, the inefficient use of health resources, a distortion in pricing behaviour and inequitable access to health care. These problems and their causes were discussed in this study; it is hoped that the following recommendations will contribute to their correction:

- The role of government in financing hospital services should be clearly defined;
- Fee schedules should be properly adjusted;
- Incomes from drugs should be effectively reduced;
- Regional health resource planning should be continuously implemented;
- The community health care system should be strengthened;
- The Zibo municipal government could commence the design and implementation of a new urban health insurance scheme, and in Nantong the health insurance scheme could be further improved;
- The fee-for-service payment system could be replaced with other kinds of payment methods.

Chapter 10

The Impact of Health Insurance Reform on Hospital Charges: A Comparison of Nantong and Zibo

Clas Rehnberg, Qingyue Meng, Ying Bian, Ning Zhuang and
Shenglan Tang

In order to control the rapid increase of hospital expenditure in urban areas, different reforms aiming at strengthening the role of the insurers as purchasers of health services have been proposed. These reforms were decided and implemented in the late 1990s as a response to some of the undesirable side effects of increasing autonomy and lack of competition in the hospital sector. This chapter analyses the impact of the recent reform of the new urban health insurance scheme by comparing Zibo and Nantong. During the late 1990s Nantong introduced new tools for controlling the providers. Following the results in Chapter 9, this chapter uses a tracer methodology where charges and utilization for two medical conditions, acute appendicitis and birth delivery, are examined and an effort is made to identify the determinants of observed differences in the performance.

The Reform of the Health Insurance System

The rapid increase of health care expenditure shown in previous chapters has forced the insurers to take action in order to curb costs and utilization. In their role as third party payers there are a number of options that could be considered for a cost containment strategy. First, there are a number of factors accountable for the increase in health care costs on both the demand and the supply side. The main factors on the demand side are changes of the demographic structure, disease pattern, socio-economic situation, and consumers' expectations. On the supply side the adoption of advanced medical technologies, drug consumption and the organization of the health systems has been emphasized (Liu and Hsiao, 1995; Hu, H., 1996; China State Council, 2000) A third party payer must deal with all these factors when a strategy for cost containment is developed. Figure 10.1 illustrates the major tools that an insurer can use with the provider and the patient in order to curb costs and utilization.

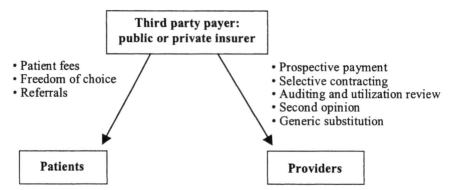

Figure 10.1 Procedures for cost control by third party payers

The measures directed at the patients aim to reduce demand by introducing fees and by other regulatory means restrict access to health services. Given the objectives of equity in access to care there are limitations on how far these measures could be used. Since the early 1980s, direct user charges have been the major source of financing for public hospitals, accounting for 90–95 per cent of total hospital income at present (World Bank, 1996). There would appear to be little scope for using co-payments to reduce the rate of rise in total health expenditure. The alternative strategy is to control costs through measures directed at the providers. The most common toll is the payment mechanism, which could be of different types of open-ended or closed-ended funding. A more recent development in several countries is to incorporate the payment system in a contractual agreement which also includes items about utilization and quality of service. Reimbursement of drugs has often been restricted to cheaper generic versions when available.

The third party payers in China, mainly the GIS and LIS systems, have used different mechanisms for funding hospitals, including the use of a bonus system in order to create incentives for hospitals to provide users with advanced technologies, pharmaceuticals and other hospital services (World Bank, 1996). More recently the government has launched reforms aimed at establishing an affordable health care system in urban cities (China State Council, 2000; Liu, 2002; Hu *et al.*, 1999). As in similar attempts to contain insurance expenditures in other countries (Propper, 1996; Yip and Eggleston, 2001; Wiley, 1992), urban health insurance reform in China included cost-containment measures on both demand and supply sides. While co-payments were established for the insured, measures such as the adoption of alternative payment methods and an increased use of provider contracting were taken for health service suppliers.

The measures on the supply side aiming at cost containment follow similar insurance arrangements that have been used in both developed and developing countries. Since the mid-1980s, case-based or capitation payment methods have been intensively adopted in the USA and most European countries for constraining the rapid growth of medical expenditures (Liu, 2002; Hu *et al.*, 1999; Dranove, 1998). Health care systems based on tax financing as well as those based on insurance have been engaged in different 'managed care' reforms. The main thread in those reforms is that the payers or the purchasers have been given more powerful tools to control the providers. In Thailand, the change of the payment systems has been used for controlling expenditures in social health insurance schemes (Mills *et al.*, 2000). In addition, insurers have been given mandates to use selective contracting of providers in order to encourage competition and thereby reducing insurance expenditures (Melrick *et al.*, 1992; Propper, 1996).

Few studies have been conducted in China to examine the health insurance effect on hospital expenditure containment. In those studies, several methodological limitations were identified, including possible changes in case mix and service quality after the reform, and the 'insurance effect on users' which means the insured would ask for more hospital services and drugs prior to the reform with anticipation of a reduced future benefit package (Yip and Eggleston, 2001; Wang, 1998; Wang and Wang, 1999; Cai, 2000). The latter would result in a sharp reduction in hospital expenses during a period immediately after the reform was implemented. This study is an effort to use data from the two cities and try to assess the effect of the urban health insurance reform. The purpose is to examine the impact of the reform on hospital charges by comparing the evolution of hospital charges between two cities, one with and one without reform, and identifying determinants for the changes identified. The chapter gives a more detailed analysis of the development of costs and utilization shown in Chapter 9 by using the tracer methodology.

Methodology

Data and Methods

The study was conducted in the two cities, Zibo and Nantong. Prior to 1997 both cities had traditional insurance systems based on the GIS and LIS structure. In Nantong the implementation of a health insurance reform in 1997 merged the different insurance plans into a single insurer for payment to providers and encouraged competition in the hospital sector. The difference in the health insurance arrangements between the two cities is part of the findings and will be presented in the results section.

Two disease conditions were chosen for a more specific analysis. Using the background information on the aims of the study and the health insurance reform, a medical expert panel selected acute appendicitis and normal childbirth to be the tracer conditions. The rationales for selecting acute appendicitis included: relatively clear diagnosis and treatment protocol for acute appendicitis that has been relatively standardized across health providers; factors which would support the assumption that hospital spending on these cases should be similar in the two cities; and the fact that there are enough appendicitis cases available in county and municipal hospitals for the purpose of sampling. The main reasons for selecting normal childbirth were that its service procedure is similar from one case to another in both cities and the incidence of childbirth in hospitals was adequate for sampling.

Hospital and health insurance documents were reviewed for comparing major variables between Zibo and Nantong relating to hospital charges, including financial incentives for hospitals and their staff and the differences in health insurance arrangements. Hospital charges in this study refer to the total medical bills presented by the hospital to its payers, either the patients (users) or insurers, including medical services and drug charges. The insured and insurers share the charges according to pre-established co-payment rates.

Data were collected from patient medical records for the two tracer conditions, reviews of hospital and health insurance documents, interviews with policy-makers and focus group discussions with hospital staff. Patient medical records kept in hospitals are the original activity and financial files for each episode of in-patient care. Hospital expenditures for each service item for the in-patient are attached to the records. Those records are relatively reliable compared to other types of hospital file such as monthly accounting reports. Basic social and demographic characteristics of the patients are registered in these records, permitting the analysis of hospital charges by patient groups.

Hospital charges were used in this study to reflect both hospital costs and expenditures. This could be a problem if charges differ from costs or expenditures. For example if hospitals charge private-paying patients with higher prices after reimbursement from the social health insurance plans (cost shifting), as suggested in studies in the USA (Dranove, 1998; Hay, 1983; Hadley and Feder, 1985; Rice *et al.*, 1996). While those studies were not consistent with the conclusion of the existence of cost shifting, they agreed some preconditions for the occurrence of cost shifting, including insensitivity of the private-paying patients to changes in prices and non-existence of competition between hospitals in the medical market. Without those preconditions, prices charged to insured and uninsured patients are thought of as a reflection of their respective costs and expenditures. The majority of the income for hospitals in China comes from out-of-pocket payments by the uninsured. The China National Health Services Survey data showed that the demand for medical care from the uninsured patients was sensitive to a rise in price (Centre for Health Statistics and Information, 1998). In addition, competition between hospitals, especially in urban cities with a surplus of hospital resources (hospital bed occupancy rate being 50–70 per cent on average for county and higher-level hospitals during 1990s), has been strong over the past two decades (Xue *et al.*, 1999). Therefore, there is little reason to conclude that there was cost shifting where the cost-constraint reform was implemented.

In addition to the tracer study based on medical records and administrative data, a number of key informant interviews were conducted. The purpose of the qualitative study was to explore the hospitals' behaviour in response to the arrangements of urban health insurance schemes and to provide supplementary information to the investigations of the quantitative data.

The Selection of Patient Medical Records, Interviewees and Participants in Focus Group Discussions

Within municipalities such as Zibo and Nantong, county and municipal general hospitals are the dominant health providers to the insured. Township and lower health facilities rarely provide services for the insured. In total there were 33 general hospitals in Nantong, from which one municipal hospital and two county hospitals were randomly selected using systematic sampling. In Zibo one municipal and two county hospitals were randomly selected from a total of 26 general hospitals. All hospitals selected in both cities were contracted by health insurance schemes.

Patient medical records for the two conditions were selected for 1995 and 1999. These years were chosen as Nantong implemented the new insurance scheme in mid-1997, and it was believed that the behaviour of both health providers and the insured in providing and demanding hospital services would be more stable two years before or after its implementation. For example, the insurance effect on users mentioned in the above section could be well controlled.

For acute appendicitis all patient medical records for these two years were collected, and for normal childbirth all records within the first three months from the beginning of each year were collected. The cases were classified into three groups: out-of-pocket users, GIS-covered patients and LIS-covered patients (users). Those three payer-groups reflected the major types of payers in urban areas at the time of the investigation. The numbers of cases and their classification are presented in Table 10.1.

Table 10.1 Number of cases of appendicitis and childbirth by user groups

User group	Zibo		Nantong	
	1995	1999	1995	1999
Acute appendicitis				
Out-of-pocket	124 (68%)	140 (76%)	134 (62%)	243 (89%)
GIS patients	26 (14%)	26 (14%)	57 (26%)	19 (7%)
LIS patients	32 (18%)	19 (10%)	25 (12%)	10 (4%)
Total	182	185	216	272
Childbirth				
Out-of-pocket	309 (70%)	383 (85%)	214 (55%)	290 (85%)
GIS patients	97 (22%)	45 (10%)	80 (21%)	39 (11%)
LIS patients	36 (8%)	21 (5%)	93 (24%)	12 (4%)
Total	442	449	387	341

The selection of patients from the three groups is stable over time for both sites and tracers. There is a slight increase of the out-of-pocket users for both tracers, especially in Nantong. The interviews were contacted for two groups. Two health officials responsible for the hospital and health insurance management from each of the cities and the Director from the Nantong Health Insurance Administrative

Centre were interviewed as key informants. Zibo had no separate government authority responsible for health insurance. A group of hospital managers, department heads, and professionals in each city (six to eight in each group) was organized for discussions.

Data Collection

A guideline was developed including a question list and indicators such as basic case characteristics (age, sex, health insurance status and occupation), health status of the in-patients on discharge and the hospital charges on service items. For the key informant interviews and focus group discussions, semi-structured question sheets were prepared which covered questions. These included: the features of the hospitals' cost-containment measures in the two cities; what would be the reform impact of urban health insurance on hospital behaviour in providing services; and how the current health insurance schemes facilitated an achievement of the cost-containment objective. The key researchers conducted the interviews and mediated the focus group discussions.

Question sheets were prepared for collecting general information from related hospital documents. Major variables included government financial inputs to the hospitals, financial incentive mechanisms operating in hospitals and the volume of the hospitals' assets. The policy documents for health insurance were collected in both cities and reviewed to identify policies related to fund management, payment method, co-payment rates and contractual relationships between insurers and health providers.

Data Analysis

Data from the medical records were used to analyse quantitatively the relationship between changes of hospital charges and their explanatory factors. The analysis was performed with comparative descriptive statistics and through a model which was set up and tested with multiple regression analysis. For supplementing the quantitative analysis, data from the interviews and focus group discussions were transcribed and analysed in relation to the themes studied. For comparing differences in hospital charges per case by category, hospital services were classified into five groups based on the hospital accounting system issued by China's Ministries of Finance and Health in 1999 (Ministry of Finance and Ministry of Health, 1999):

- Drugs
- Bed
- Surgical operation
- Non-pharmacological treatment
- Others.

Non-pharmacological treatment and 'others' consist of a number of fee items. The former includes hospital professional services, nursing service and blood and oxygen supplies. The latter includes laboratory tests, food, office supplies and air conditioner charges. Monetary values for the hospital charges in 1995 were adjusted to the values in 1999 with the consumption price indices in the two cities (using the price index in 1999 as 100, the price indices in Zibo and Nantong in 1995 were 91.7 and 91.9) (Zibo Bureau of Statistics, 2000; Nantong Bureau of Statistics, 2000).

Results

This section presents the major findings of the study. The first part describes the major differences in the insurance arrangements between the two cities. In the second part a comparison is made of hospital charges and their growth trends before and after the health insurance reform in Nantong. In the last section, the daily charges of various service categories are compared between the two cities. In the appendix to this chapter an explanatory model is set up to identify the factors influencing the outcome of the reform.

Financial Incentives and Insurance Arrangements

On 1 April 1997, Nantong began implementing the new urban health insurance reforms, while the urban health insurance system implemented in Zibo maintained the traditional GIS and LIS models. Hence, from 1997 on, Zibo and Nantong operated with different models of urban health insurance. The differences in health insurance arrangements between Zibo and Nantong from 1997 were characterized by the number of health insurers, payment methods, co-payment rates of hospital charges, and the introduction of an essential drug list (see Table 10.2).

The new insurance arrangement has given the insurer side some new tools to be used for purchasing and reimbursement for health services. The integration of insurers into one body put them in a more powerful position towards the providers. The selection of providers and the payment system transfer some risk to the providers and give incentives for efficient delivery of services. There are also a number of changes on the demand side such as higher co-payments, restriction on the use of drugs and freedom of choice of providers.

The financing system of the two cities did not show any major changes over time. Direct user fees and insurance payments were the major sources of revenue for all the sample hospitals. In 1999, 95 per cent of the revenue in Zibo's hospitals and 94 per cent of the revenue in Nantong's hospitals came from such charges. Still, for GIS and LIS beneficiaries, a large part is reimbursed retrospectively. The share of direct government budgets in total hospital revenue accounted for a mere 5–6 per cent in the two cities.

In Nantong a system with fixed payments for in-patient days was used, and the insurers were still receiving an itemization of charges from each hospital. Between 1997 and 1999, a major change was introduced in Nantong's health insurance arrangement where the average LOS and readmission rates were regulated as a supplementary measure to the payment method. One notable change in Zibo was that, after 1996, childbirth covered by LIS was reimbursed at a fixed rate by many businesses. In interviews, the Director of the Nantong Health Insurance Management Centre recognized that one of their tough tasks was to control hospital charges. The most commonly repeated reason why urban health insurance reform was not introduced in Zibo was that it was very hard to collect the insurance premiums fund from some enterprises, since the profitable enterprises were not willing to join, while the loss-making enterprises were not able to afford the payment of insurance premium for their employees and retirees.

Table 10.2 Differences in urban health insurance arrangements between Zibo and Nantong

Features of the insurance schemes	Zibo	Nantong
Number of insurers	Multiple insurers (separate institutions).	Single insurer.
Fund management and allocation	Funds managed by separate institutions.	Funds were divided into two parts: health account and risk pooling. Half went to health account and half went to the risk-pooling fund.
Selection of providers	One or two providers for out-patient and in-patient services.	Patients chose out-patient providers themselves; 4–5 in-patient providers contracted.
Payment method	Mainly fee-for-service. From 1996, many businesses set a fixed reimbursement rate for childbirth.	Fixed prices per out-patient visit and per in-patient day (irrespective of diagnosis). Rates are adjusted once a year mainly according to inflation.
Co-payment by the insured	Co-payment rate was set by each insurer, approximately 5% of hospital charges below CNY5,000 and 10% above CNY5,000.	Percentages vary with expenditure level per treatment episode, 5% of co-payment rate below CNY5,000 in expenses and 16% above CNY5,000.
Contractual relations	Contracting was not used for many insurers.	Strict contractual regulations between insurer and health providers.
Drug use	No restriction on prescribing.	Coverage restricted to essential drug list. Drugs are included in the fixed payment per in-patient day.

Hospital service quality in both cities increased over the last decade and there were no identified differences in service quality between the two cities in 1995 and 1999 (Meng *et al.*, 2001). Health officials interviewed from both cities thought that the escalation of hospital costs was a major problem over the past years. They attributed this mainly to the current hospital financial policy and the lack of strong control of third parties over hospitals' charging behaviour, which consequently led to the provision of unnecessary hospital services. The interviewees recognized three measures that were proposed for controlling hospital expenditures in urban areas: regional health planning, re-establishment of the community health care system and reforming the urban health insurance system. Zibo introduced regional health planning from the early 1990s. The effectiveness of this initiative in Zibo was neither documented nor supported by the Zibo health officials interviewed. Nantong did not introduce regional health planning during the study period. The community health care system was not effectively re-established in either city when the study was conducted.

Characteristics of the Cases

A change in the insurance system might give the insurers and the providers' incentives to avoid patient with certain characteristics. It is therefore important to consider changes in the patient workload over time. The health insurance status for the cases was listed in Table 10.1. In Table 10.3 the sex, age and length of stay per case and their comparisons between both cities are shown.

Table 10.3 Characteristics and average charges of the cases, comparisons between both cities

Variables	1995			1999		
	Zibo	Nantong	*t-stat.*	Zibo	Nantong	*t-stat.*
Acute appendicitis						
Sex: male %	34.6	46.8	$6.01^a (\chi^2)$	42.1	45.2	$0.04 (\chi^2)$
Age (years)	33.2	32.6	0.382	33.8	34.0	−0.099
LOS (days)	9.8	8.2	4.463^b	8.8	7.5	4.356^b
Childbirth						
Age (years)	27.5	25.5	8.474^b	27.7	26.0	7.753^b
LOS (days)	4.57	7.37	$−18.320^b$	5.19	6.43	$−5.704^b$

[a]Statistically significant at 5% level; [b]Statistically significant at 1% level

Significant differences were found for acute appendicitis cases in sex structure in 1995 with greater proportion of males in Nantong and in average LOS, with a longer stay in Zibo for both years. There were no significant differences in ages between the two cities for acute appendicitis. For childbirth, significant differences in age (older in Zibo) and average LOS (longer in Nantong) were found between both cities for both years. For childbirth, the average age of the cases in Nantong was higher in 1999 than that in 1995 ($P<0.05$). The LOS for childbirth increased in Zibo and decreased in Nantong in 1999 ($P<0.01$). The differences in charges per patient are presented in Figure 10.2.

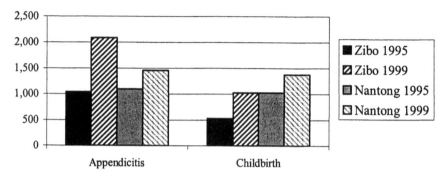

Figure 10.2 Comparison of hospital expenses per case (CNY) between Zibo and Nantong

There are a number of observations to be made from these figures. In 1995, there were no statistical differences in hospital charges per acute appendicitis case between Zibo and Nantong. In 1999, hospital charge per case was significantly higher in Zibo than in Nantong. Zibo's hospital charge per acute appendicitis case in 1999 was 43 per cent higher than that in Nantong. However, for normal childbirth Nantong showed prior to the reform in 1995 a rate that was 94 per cent more expensive than that in Zibo. The charges per childbirth were still higher in Nantong than in Zibo in 1999, but the gap fell to 34 per cent, still a significant difference.

As the level of expenditure is influenced by local circumstances as is the level of costs etc., it is also of interest to consider the growth rate of expenditures. Hospital charges per case of both acute appendicitis and childbirth increased significantly from 1995 to 1999 in the two cities. Growth rates of hospital charges on acute appendicitis between 1995 and 1999 were 101 per cent in Zibo and 41 per cent in Nantong. Also for childbirth Zibo showed a higher growth rate between 1995 and 1999 than Nantong, 94 per cent and 34 per cent respectively. Hence, considering the growth rates, it is obvious that the new system in Nantong has put some restrictions on the previous cost escalation.

Hospital Charges and Growth Rates by User Groups

Another uncertainty over the insurance reform is the effect on different user groups. As the different insurance schemes only cover a smaller share of the population in urban areas, the impact for the uninsured paying user fees must be considered. Table 10.4 presents the growth rates of hospital charges for acute appendicitis and childbirth by user groups from 1995 to 1999.

Overall, we can observe a slower growth rate in Nantong than in Zibo. In Zibo, the growth rate for appendicitis is higher for LIS patients, whereas childbirth charge per LIS case was significantly lower than that of out-of-pocket and GIS cases. In Nantong, the growth rate of childbirth charges per out-of-pocket case was higher than that of GIS users, but not LIS users. In total, it is difficult to see a pattern and there is no indication of a marked strategy for cost shifting.

Table 10.4 Growth rates (percentage change) of hospital charges for acute appendicitis and childbirth by insured groups between 1995 and 1999

User group	Acute appendicitis (%)	Childbirth (%)
Zibo		
Out-of-pocket	98	116
GIS patients	119	91
LIS patients	124	49
Total	101	94
Nantong		
Out-of-pocket	36	40
GIS patients	38	27
LIS patients	42	46
Total	41	34

Another way of analysing the effects for different patient groups is to study the difference in charges per patient between Zibo and Nantong. Table 10.5 presents the means of hospital charges per case of acute appendicitis and childbirth and their comparisons between the two cities. In 1995, significant differences in hospital charges of acute appendicitis between Zibo and Nantong were found only in the out-of-pocket user group, where Nantong had a higher rate. In 1999, hospital charges per acute appendicitis case were significantly higher in the three user groups in Zibo than in Nantong. For both insured and uninsured users, Nantong's hospital charges per case of childbirth were higher than Zibo's in 1995. Nantong's hospital charges per case of out-of-pocket and LIS childbirth were still significantly higher than those of Zibo in 1999.

Table 10.5 Means and standard deviations of hospital charges (CNY) per case and their comparisons between Zibo and Nantong

User group	1995			1999		
	Zibo	Nantong	*t-stat.*	Zibo	Nantong	*t-stat.*
Acute appendicitis						
Out-of-pocket	953	1,058	−2.139[a]	1,885	1,437	7.324[b]
GIS patients	1,276	1,112	1.431	2,795	1,529	4.440[b]
LIS patients	1,161	1,261	−0.772	2,597	1,786	2.081[a]
Childbirth						
Out-of-pocket	458	969	−28.812[b]	991	1,361	−11.320[b]
GIS patients	718	1,127	−10.33[b]	1,371	1,435	−0.470
LIS patients	633	1,062	−7.653[b]	947	1,550	−3.999[b]

[a]Statistically significant at 5% level; [b]Statistically significant at 1% level.

In 1999 in Zibo, both GIS and LIS acute appendicitis patients spent more than out-of-pocket patients did ($P<0.001$), representing 38–48 per cent higher expense. In Nantong, significant differences in hospital charges between out-of-pocket and LIS acute appendicitis cases existed with 24 per cent more spending for LIS patients than for out-of-pocket patients in 1999 ($P<0.05$). In 1999, charges per GIS-covered childbirth were higher than those of out-of-pocket and LIS-covered childbirth ($P<0.001$). In Nantong, there were no significant differences in childbirth charges among the user groups in 1999.

Nantong's health insurance manager and health officials reflected that there was a positive impact from the reformed health insurance scheme on the control of hospital charges. They identified three reasons. First, the power of a single insurer within a city is much greater than it was before unification. The single insurer is regarded as being in a better position to control behaviour of both the providers and the insured in prescribing and utilization of hospital services. Second, hospitals had to control increases in charges, or the health insurer would not contract them. Lastly, it became easier after implementation of the reform to regulate hospitals' charges with the new payment method and the essential drug list. During discussion, hospital staff in Nantong said that they had felt the pressure to contain hospital charges after the reform and that the quality and prices of hospital services were the two most important measures for them to compete for the insurance contracts (in the appendix to this chapter a quantitative model for determining the factors influencing the changes in hospital charges is presented).

Changes in Hospital Charges Per Case by Service Categories

Hospital charges are laid down for different types of service delivered by the hospitals. The major service categories analysed in this section are drug-treatment, non-pharmacological treatment and surgical operations. In addition to this there are two other charges for beds and other services. In this section we show the detailed changes in charges per service category for acute appendicitis to illustrate how hospitals have achieved savings. All service categories except bed fees in 1999 were significantly different between the two cities for both years. Higher drug expenses and surgical operation fees were the main contributors to higher total charges per case in Nantong over Zibo in 1995 (Figure 10.3).

It is obvious that the lower increase rate of charges in Nantong is mainly for drug expenditure and non-pharmacological treatment, whereas charges for surgical operations have continued to increase. The direction of differences in drug charges per case reversed from 1995 to 1999 in the two cities. In Zibo, from 1995 to 1999, charges for drug and non-pharmacological treatment increased by CNY446 and CNY453 per case, with growth rates of 140 per cent and 98 per cent. Increase of charges for those two items accounted for 86 per cent of the total increase of charge per case in Zibo from 1995 to 1999. Over the same period in Nantong, charges per case for drugs remained at the same level while non-pharmacological treatment increased by CNY144 (45 per cent). The charge per patient for surgical operations was still higher in Nantong than in Zibo, and the increase rate was also higher, 97 per cent in Nantong compared with 43 per cent in Zibo.

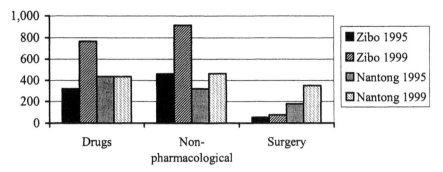

Figure 10.3 Hospital charges per service category (CNY), Zibo and Nantong, 1995–9

The hospital staff in the discussion groups from both cities admitted that drug charges were their main financial source of cost recovery. Hospitals can generally earn 20–30 per cent mark-up rates on drug sales. They argued that the costs of operating some services, such as medical consultation, could not be fully recovered because of low prices set by the government. Making some profit from drug sales could compensate for losses of this kind in other areas. Some hospital managers also indicated that GIS and LIS patients usually asked for more drugs, not necessarily for the insured themselves, but for uninsured family members or relatives. Both policy-makers and hospital staff from Nantong emphasized the importance of implementing the essential drug list for controlling drug expenses in the reformed insurance scheme.

Discussion

The changes in Chinese health care financing that took place in the 1980s made the hospitals dependent on revenues from direct and indirect user charges and gave health providers a considerable autonomy to allocate surpluses. In the original individual-institution-based GIS and LIS models in China, the insurers were actually production-dominated businesses or government agencies rather than pure insurance management entities. They had neither adequate administrative skill to control hospitals, nor did their individual institutional health funds have the negotiating power to effectively regulate hospital behaviour. By introducing reforms based on the unification of several hundreds or thousands of insurers into a single insurer, the pooling of health insurance funds from all institutions in the city provides a stronger position for negotiating prices and service quality with the hospitals. Zwanziger and Melnick (1988) have stressed the importance of relative power between health providers and purchasers in hospital prices in the USA. In the Netherlands, Lieverdink (2001) observed that the insurers' power to force health providers to improve efficiency has been reduced because of competition between sickness funds. This study supports that the establishment of a single insurer in a given city is an essential difference between the old and new health insurance schemes.

The health insurance reform based on a single insurer implemented in Nantong in 1997 appears to have been successful in reducing the rates of growth of hospital charges, which were far lower in Nantong than in Zibo for all user groups, even for the out-of-pocket paying majority. The average LOS was also reduced in Nantong, which is an important factor determining hospital charges. Charges on drugs and non-pharmacological treatments for acute appendicitis increased more rapidly for the city without reform than for the city with reform.

Both quantitative and qualitative analysis suggest that the urban health insurance reform was likely to be the major reason for the reduced rate of growth of hospital charges in Nantong. By comparing the differences in insurance arrangements between the two cities, it is shown that the charge containment may result from four types of reform measures implemented:

- The establishment of a single insurer across the city;
- The encouragement of hospital competition for insurance contracts;
- The implementation of a fixed-charge payment method;
- The restriction of drug coverage based on an essential drug list.

The study does not highlight a particular tool as more important than others. The development of the length of stay could illustrate the need to work with several tools simultaneously. From 1995 to 1999, the average LOS was reduced by one day for all patients in China, similar to our finding for the two cities (Ministry of Health, 2002). It was also found that the insured population in China had a longer average LOS than did the uninsured for a given health condition (Tu *et al.*, 2002). In our study, the fixed-charge payment method used in Nantong seems to control the charge per in-patient day in those cases where hospitalization was required. This method therefore provides an incentive for hospitals to prolong the LOS in order to generate more revenues from each in-patient. For this reason, the Nantong insurance authority issued supplementary measures to the payment method for controlling LOS and readmission rates, as pointed out by the insurance manager. This highlights the need for payment reforms to be accompanied by other supplementary measures, to compensate for undesirable incentives.

Our results are not unambiguous and there might be other external factors influencing the costs and expenses. One example is the longer average LOS for childbirth in Nantong compared with Zibo. Differences in average LOS between the two cities and over time might have two possible explanations. First, the average LOS of childbirth might be more influenced by users' income level than by other factors. The one-child policy in urban China could make couples place service quality and safety as their top priority over cost. Parents or health professionals may view a longer stay in hospitals as better and safer for the baby. It was reported that in wealthy areas childbirth at tertiary hospitals, bypassing township, and county hospitals, has increased (Ministry of Health, 1999). Parents in Nantong who are wealthier than those in Zibo may ask for longer hospital stay. However, because the above explanation does not clarify why Nantong's average

LOS decreased between 1995 and 1999, another reason may be that health insurance arrangement might have some impact on LOS. A finding in Zibo that LIS childbirths spent much less than GIS childbirths after the change to the reimbursement method for LIS childbirth supports the latter explanation.

Drug consumption played an important role in determining the level of hospital charges in China (World Bank, 1996; Hu and Gong, 1999) The slower growth rate of drug charges in Nantong may be attributable to the adoption of an essential drug list and the fixed-charge payment method. The drug list excluded some expensive and imported drugs that limited the scope of drugs for doctors to prescribe. In addition, the insured must bear the expenses themselves of drugs not included in the list, which could constrain their demand. Second, the fixed-charge payment method imposes more pressure than a fee-for-service payment system on hospitals to control expenses. Because drug expenses accounted for a large proportion of the total medical expenses, hospitals could put drugs as one of the priorities in expense control, in order not to exceed the unit reimbursement from the insurer. In addition, when net revenues from drug prescriptions are less than that from the provision of hospital professional services (Meng *et al.*, 2002), it would be reasonable for hospitals to reduce the proportion of the drug expense in total unit charges. Given the findings in other studies that unnecessary prescriptions accounted for a large proportion of the total drug expenses (Hu and Gong, 1999), it seems possible to control drug expenses without affecting the use of necessary drugs.

Differences in the evolution of charges for non-pharmacological treatments between the two cities after the health insurance reform may be directly related to their different payment methods. Non-pharmacological treatment consists of a number of fee items, unlike fees for surgical operations, which is a single fee item in the fee schedule. Because hospitals only report the total expenses in the category of non-pharmacological treatment rather than itemizing each expense when patients are discharged, under a fee-for-service payment system, charges for these combined fee items can be more distorted than in itemized expenses. A fixed-charge payment method that sets pre-established limits for each unit of out-patient visits and in-patient days, irrespective of the amount and value of items and services consumed, can help contain the controllable expenses. While drugs charges seem to be sensitive to changes in the insurance arrangement, some of the non-drug items are less sensitive. This accounts especially for the charges for surgical operations for acute appendicitis, which shows a dramatic increase in Nantong. This explains the difficulties in controlling the internal medical decision-making process in hospitals.

Although two tracer conditions were used to try to control the severity of health conditions among cases and between the two cities, and to permit the calculation and comparison of detailed pre- and post-reform charges, this study has several limitations. One limitation is the limited number of insured cases for analysis, which may influence the stability of the results. In addition, one should be cautious regarding the ability of the two conditions to represent in-patient care in general. The two conditions studied account for a small portion of the total hospital in-patient care and expenses, which makes it difficult to generalize the conclusions. Still, the results could very well serve as a well-founded hypothesis for tests based on more extensive and comprehensive data material. The problems in the use of the conditions could be overcome by using larger numbers of cases and conditions in future research. In this study, the trends followed by the hospital charges were compared. However, it has not been possible to quantify the effects on those trends owing to the retrospective nature of the data.

Conclusion

The introduction of the new urban insurance system shows some positive impact on hospital costs and efficiency. The study also shows that it is necessary to provide insurers with tools and instruments to become an efficient purchaser of health services. Achieving the effective control of hospital expenses will be a key determinant for the success of the reform, since the expansion of the coverage of insurance systems to a greater part of the population can only occur with an effective cost-containment arrangement. The health insurance reform in the pilot cities studied demonstrated the positive effects of containing the growth of hospital charges for both conditions. It is also important to note that this effect has not been achieved by shifting charges to other non-insured patients. The most important elements in the insurance arrangement influencing hospital charges included the establishment of a single insurance scheme within the municipality, adoption of an alternative payment system replacing fee-for-service payment method and the introduction of an essential drug list. The combined effects of these measures, rather than a single measure in the health insurance arrangement, is likely to be more effective in controlling hospital charges. Overall, it is important that those insurers are given the right to act on behalf of the premium payers, that is, the employers and the employees.

Appendix:
Regression Analysis of Factors Influencing Hospital Charges in Both Conditions

Multiple regression analysis (Stepwise) was used together with the data from patient records. As the arrangement of health insurance in 1999 differed from that in 1995 for Nantong and childbirth insurance reimbursement was also changed in 1999 for Zibo, the models were run separately for the two cities and each of the years. Since the patients' occupations had high correlation with their health insurance status, it was not included in the model.

$$AC_{cy} = \beta_1 + \beta_2 Sex_{cy} + \beta_3 Age_{cy} + \beta_4 Insu_{cy} + \beta_5 LOS_{cy}$$

where

  ß = Coefficient
  AC = average charge per in-patient (CNY)
  Sex = Sex of the patients, applicable for acute appendicitis only (0 = male, 1 = female)
  Age = Age of the patients (years)(expected positive coefficient)
  Insu = Insurance status of the patients (0 = out-of-pocket, 1 = GIS and LIS) (Expected positive coefficient)
  LOS = Hospital length of stay of the patients (days) (expected positive coefficient)
  c = cities (Zibo or Nantong)
  y = year (1995 or 1999)

Differences in hospital charges per case and hospital charges by service categories over time and between the two cities were compared using student T-test statistics. One-way ANOVA statistics were used to test the differences in hospital charges among the user groups and Chi-square test was to compare the gender compositions of the acute appendicitis cases. Table 10.6 shows the results for determining the factors influencing hospital charge per case.

For each case of acute appendicitis, health insurance status was significantly associated with the hospital charges in Zibo in 1999 and in Nantong in 1995, in which GIS- and LIS-covered patients spent more than out-of-pocket patients. After the reform in Nantong, health insurance status was no longer a variable significantly influencing hospital charges per case. The average LOS was significant for hospital charges per case in all regressions for acute appendicitis. Age in all regressions but Zibo in 1999 was significant for changes in hospital charges, with more spending on older patients. Sex influence was found in Nantong in 1999 only.

For childbirth, insurance status was influential in 1995 for both cities, with greater spending for GIS- and LIS-covered childbirths than for out-of-pocket ones. In 1999, a significant association was found between health insurance status and charges in Zibo, but not in Nantong. As with acute appendicitis, average LOS was influential in all regressions for childbirth. Age was not found to be significant for hospital charges for childbirth.

Table 10.6 Multiple regression results (dependent variable: hospital charge per case)

Variable	Zibo 1995		Zibo 1999		Nantong 1995		Nantong 1999	
	Coeff.	t-stat.	Coeff.	t-stat.	Coeff.	t-stat.	Coeff.	t-stat.
Acute appendicitis								
Sex	73.0	1.19	−13.3	−0.13	−47.1	−1.26	−88.2	−1.98[a]
	(61.1)		(104.8)		(37.4)		(44.7)	
Age	4.6	2.17[a]	3.06	0.91	6.4	5.02[b]	8.6	6.33[b]
	(2.1)		(3.3)		(1.3)		(1.4)	
Insurance	79.0	1.21	589.0	4.83[b]	99.9	2.59[b]	32.0	0.66
	(65.3)		(121.9)		(38.5)		(72.5)	
LOS	62.5	8.98[b]	130.9	9.18[b]	75.5	12.01[b]	86.7	9.88[b]
	(7.0)		(14.3)		(6.3)		(8.8)	
Constant	203.6	2.01[a]	697.9	4.37[b]	257.0	3.88[b]	563.8	7.20[b]
	(101.0)		(159.8)		(66.3)		(78.3)	
N	182		185		216		272	
Adjusted R^2	0.364		0.441		0.493		0.372	
Prob.>F	0.000		0.000		0.000		0.000	
Childbirth								
Age	0.28	0.142	−5.18	−0.85	2.72	0.52	2.79	0.40
	(1.99)		(6.1)		(5.2)		(6.9)	
Insurance	215.6	12.74[b]	164.3	2.87[b]	113.5	4.65[b]	13.5	0.25
	(16.9)		(57.2)		(24.4)		(53.7)	
LOS	50.4	4.04[b]	50.0	8.89[b]	4.9	4.6[b]	124.6	12.82[b]
	(4.0)		(5.6)		(10.7)		(9.7)	
Constant	225.9	3.691[b]	867.7	5.07[b]	516.6	3.69[b]	500.3	2.51[a]
	(61.2)		(175.1)		(139.9)		(199.5)	
N	442		449		387		341	
Adjusted R^2	0.448		0.179		0.262		0.330	
Prob.>F	0.000		0.000		0.000		0.000	

Note: Standard errors in parentheses
[a]Statistically significant at 5% level; [b]Statistically significant at 1% level

Chapter 11

Conclusions and Recommendations

Gerald Bloom, Qingyue Meng and Shenglan Tang

Conclusions

This chapter brings together the conclusions and policy recommendations of the study. It draws heavily on discussions at workshops in each city, a national workshop for researchers and government officials and a one-day meeting of senior researchers and officials of a number of provincial health departments at the annual meeting of the Chinese Social Medicine Association. It highlights the issues that the participants at these meetings considered to be important.

The study took place in two out of China's 311 cities with more than 200,000 people. Both are in the more prosperous part of the country. One has to be cautious in applying the findings to China as a whole. None the less, participants at the national meetings agreed that the problems and structural constraints to change that the two in-depth snapshots revealed were relevant to most other cities. This section organizes the conclusions in terms of changing health care needs, health finance and utilization, and the organization and management of health services.

Changing Health Care Needs

Nantong and Zibo illustrate the dramatic demographic and epidemiological transition that China has experienced over the past two decades. They have ageing populations and the top six causes of death are non-communicable diseases. The rapidly growing number of elderly people is an important source of increased demand for health services. They tend to have higher prevalence of chronic disease. Also, hospital care during the last year of a person's life tends to account for a significant share of total health care costs.

Another factor contributing to the changing pattern of health care needs is the growing number of urban poor with higher than average levels of acute and chronic illness. Also many rural people are migrating to the city. They are younger and healthier than average, but they tend to have a higher incidence of infectious disease, associated with their living conditions in the cities and in the rural areas from which they originate.

Health Finance and Utilization

The study found that access to health care was influenced by household income and health insurance status. Employees of profitable enterprises and their families used health services more than employees of loss-making enterprises.

The elderly had quite different experiences in the two cities. They had higher incomes in Nantong. Also 92 per cent of our sample of elderly in Nantong had health insurance, compared with 39 per cent in Zibo. Despite the differences in insurance coverage, levels of utilization were similar in the two cities. This is partly due to the greater availability of public and private primary care facilities in Zibo. Residents of Nantong made much greater use of referral hospitals for ambulatory care. Elderly residents of Zibo bore a higher burden of health care costs themselves, particularly when they had a chronic disease.

Few poor families had health insurance. However, they reported a higher than average number of health problems. They commonly treated themselves. In Zibo, they also used public and private clinics. The team interviewed a number of people who had experienced great difficulty in paying for health care. This is clearly a major problem for many families.

People with chronic disease bore a heavy financial burden, particularly if they had no insurance. Zibo residents with a chronic disease, but without insurance, reported median expenditure of 17.2 per cent of annual household income on health care. This reflects the rapid rise in the cost of out-patient care: three-fold in Zibo and almost four-fold in Nantong during the 1990s. Although average incomes rose, many were left behind. This contributed to the increasing financial barriers to access to care.

Nantong introduced a new health insurance scheme in 1997. A disproportionate number of enterprises with an older workforce joined the scheme, since it made it easier for them to provide benefits to their retirees. Enterprises with a younger workforce refused to join and the scheme was experiencing financial problems at the time of the study. Subsequently, the scheme decreased contribution rates and reduced benefits for out-patient services. The government agreed to pay for the health benefits to which a small number of elderly are entitled because of previous service in the liberation army or high political status. As a result of these changes, many more companies joined the scheme and its financial situation improved. It is difficult to predict how the rising number of very old beneficiaries will affect its financial viability over time.

The Nantong Health Insurance Scheme allows beneficiaries to make claims on the pooled resources for only in-patient care and six chronic diseases. Patients pay for other out-patient services from the limited allocation to their individual accounts and in cash. This puts a heavy financial burden on the families of people with chronic disease.

Organization and Management of Health Services

The study focused on hospital services, which account for a high proportion of total health expenditure in the cities. The organization and management of these services changed considerably during the 1990s. The productivity of services declined substantially. This was due to increases in cost of services and falls in utilization. During the late 1990s the expansion in the number of beds and in the number of health workers slowed down, but hospitals continued to procure high-technology medical equipment.

During the early 1990s hospitals in both cities introduced a responsibility system to improve performance. The incomes of departments and individual workers were influenced by their performance in terms of workload, quality of services, revenue generation and patient satisfaction. Efficiency declined, despite this system. The study found that hospitals did not necessarily adhere to official fee schedules. Also, doctors tended to provide more diagnostic tests and prescribe more drugs for patients with health insurance. The researchers had the impression that hospitals met their revenue targets by raising prices and encouraging a costly style of medical care. The emphasis on revenue generation was closely related to the fact that government funding accounted for as little as 5 per cent of a hospital's total budget.

The study found that Nantong's reformed health insurance scheme succeeded in slowing down the increase in hospital costs. It attributed this to a combination of the enforcement of an essential drugs policy, the award of contracts to providers on a competitive basis and payment of a fixed amount per out-patient visit and in-patient day. These conclusions are based on a study of the cost of treatment of appendicitis and assisted delivery. More research is needed to assess the impact of the reforms on other kinds of treatment and identify the strategies with the greatest influence on hospital performance.

Recommendations

The discussions between the research team and participants at the end-of-project meetings generated the following recommendations.

City health departments need to strengthen their public health and preventive programmes. Recent national policy statements have underlined the responsibility of local governments to finance and provide these services. However, at the time this chapter was written there was little evidence of a major increase in funding of these services. Cities that have enjoyed rapid economic growth should be able to fund their own public health services; others may need financial assistance from higher levels of government.

The public health services need to adapt to changing patterns of need. The low birth rate has led to a fall in demand for maternal and child health services, while the ageing of the population has generated unmet needs for a variety of support services. The growing number of poor and socially excluded people and the large rural-to-urban migration is also creating new needs. The public health services need to strengthen their capacity to monitor for, and respond to, new needs.

Health insurance reform is the centrepiece of the government's strategy for financing urban health services. The aim should be gradually to establish compulsory basic health insurance schemes in all cities. The richer cities could supplement the basic scheme. The challenge is to convince younger workers that they will ultimately benefit from these schemes. Otherwise they will view their contributions as a tax. The schemes presently do not cover family members of employees. This works to the detriment of middle-aged and elderly women, who are more likely to be out of a job than their male counterparts. The present schemes provide only partial benefits for out-patient treatment of chronic illness. This creates a heavy burden on some households and could encourage more in-patient treatment. More work is needed to find ways to address this problem.

Reforms to health insurance are unlikely to succeed unless they are accompanied by changes to the service delivery system. The present heavy reliance on acute care hospitals for out-patient treatment and the care of the chronically ill is very expensive. Better primary level medical care and community support are needed. Hospital management needs to be strengthened to reverse the decline in efficiency. Special measures are needed to encourage a more rational use of diagnostic technologies and pharmaceutical products. Health insurance schemes need to improve their capacity to purchase services effectively on behalf of members and their employers. Health bureaux need to strengthen their ability to monitor and regulate health facility performance. City governments need to be more active in planning the development of their health services. The public needs more information on the options for reform and on the performance of the health system.

The rising number of elderly is creating a special challenge. Most cities will not be able to provide everyone with the kind of hospital-based health care that those with full health insurance currently enjoy. Cities need to develop alternative ways to meet the needs of the elderly by strengthening primary health care services, community support for people in their homes and nursing homes for the seriously disabled. New health insurance schemes may find it difficult to fund health care for the elderly out of insurance contributions by younger workers and their employers alone. In that case, governments will need to contribute some of the cost. Otherwise, there is a risk that health insurance schemes could lose public support.

It will be some time before everyone is fully insured. However, government can take other measures to protect the rest of the urban population. It can fund public health services and preventive programmes adequately. It can encourage the development of cost-effective out-patient facilities and monitor and regulate their performance. It can also reduce the over-prescription of drugs by ending the direct linkage between health worker income and volume of drug sales and organizing public education programmes. The government has begun to experiment with a health safety net for the poor. A lot of work needs to be done to determine the relative importance of chronic disease and acute hospitalizations and to ensure that poor people have sufficient access to essential health care.

One of the greatest challenges to city health departments is the changing nature of the populations they serve. Many localities outside city boundaries are becoming increasingly urbanized. These localities may be gradually integrated into the city. In the health sector, this will involve many issues regarding the organization and finance of public health services and the reform of insurance schemes. It will make it increasingly difficult to maintain the kinds of benefits that employees of profitable enterprises still enjoy.

Rural-to-urban migrants now constitute an important, but unknown, proportion of urban residents. Municipal governments need to take some responsibility for their health care for two reasons. First, they are tax payers and should be entitled to benefits. Also, there are good grounds on the basis of public health for including them in preventive programmes. This is certainly the case for tuberculosis and sexually transmitted infections. The importance of this issue was graphically illustrated during the SARS (Severe Acute Respiratory Syndrome) outbreak, when migrants were seen as a potential source of spread of infection to other localities. The government needs to develop more effective ways to encourage the organizations and institutions which hire migrant workers to participate in urban health insurance schemes. This raises difficult questions about whether benefits should be portable when migrants return to their rural homes. The government also needs to ensure that public health and preventive programmes cover migrants.

For the past 20 years the government has responded passively to problems that urban health services have experienced as the country has managed its transition to a market economy. These responses have enabled health facilities to remain financially viable and to improve their buildings and equipment. However, it has become clear that serious problems have emerged and urban residents are very concerned about them. Costs have risen rapidly and many people are now anxious about how they would cope with the financial cost of a serious illness. A significant number of people simply cannot get access to important medical care. The government has announced that it is giving priority to measures to tackle these problems. The major conclusion of this study is that it will require a long-term and concerted effort to overcome the structural problems that have led to the present situation.

Annex

Research Methods

This chapter presents details of the research methods used in the data collection conducted in the two study cities, Nantong and Zibo, in 1999 and 2000. The first section considers the equity study undertaken by the School of Public Health at Fudan University, the Institute of Development Studies and the University of Hamburg. The second describes the efficiency study, jointly organized by the Institute of Social Medicine and Health Policy at Shandong University and the Centre for Health Economics at the Stockholm School of Economics.

Equity Study

Data collection in the equity study included two household health surveys, a work-unit survey and qualitative studies using focus group discussions and in-depth interviews. These were designed to examine the issue of access to and financing of health services, with a special focus on the factors affecting the access of vulnerable groups.

Household Surveys

Organization of the surveys
Two household health surveys were conducted in each of the two cities. One, described as the work unit-based survey, sampled households via the previously selected enterprise or institution that employed one of their members. The other, the community-based survey, sampled households from selected areas of each city with the objective of identifying potentially 'vulnerable' households.

The work unit-based survey Work units were classified under five headings: (1) government agencies and public institutions, (2) profitable state-owned enterprises (SOEs), (3) loss-making SOEs, (4) collective enterprises (COEs), and (5) others. These were defined as follows:

1 *Government agencies and public institutions*. Workers in these institutions were covered by the Government Insurance Scheme (GIS) prior to the introduction of the health insurance reforms. The health benefits enjoyed were typically superior to those provided by enterprises.
2/3 *Profitable and loss-making SOEs*. All workers in SOEs are in principle covered by the Labour Insurance Scheme (LIS). However, the health benefits offered

vary a great deal in accordance with the economic status of the enterprise. They were therefore further classified as either profitable or loss-making.

4 *Collective enterprises.* COEs are enterprises that belong to collective institutions, such as street administrative committees, or public institutions with collective property. Some enterprises of this kind were implementing the GIS, as advised by the government, but others were not.

5 *Others.* Other enterprises include joint-venture, joint-stock, foreign-investment, and privately run. All have in general been profitable and many have developed their own health benefit packages. Some are implementing the LIS and provide similar health benefits to the SOEs. However, others provide very limited health benefits to their employees or none at all.

Community-based survey The vulnerable groups initially identified for the community-based household health survey were those living in specific categories of households: primary earner unemployed or laid off by their employer; primary earner disabled; all household members over 60; officially designated as poor; and migrant households. Because the research team found that there were only a small number of disabled in the selected communities, these households were not included in the questionnaire survey, but a number were selected for the qualitative study.

Sample size and sampling methods
Different sampling strategies were employed according to the particular features of the various populations. Adopting a variety of approaches was necessary to facilitate data collection, but implied that considerable care was required in analysis and interpretation.

Work unit-based survey The total number of households sampled in the selected institutions was 1,000. These were distributed across 20 sampled work units: two government agencies/public institutions, four profitable SOEs, six loss-making SOEs, four collective enterprises and four others. An equal number of households (50) were sampled from each work unit.

A number of criteria were used to select the enterprises for the survey:

1 Of the two government agencies and public institutions, one should be a government agency, such as a municipal health bureau, and the other should be a public institution, such as a school or hospital.
2 The four profitable SOEs should be sampled from the highest or nearly highest profit-making SOEs. Two should be covered by the new health insurance scheme, if the new scheme existed in the study city.
3 The six loss-making SOEs should be operating more or less normally in spite of their economic status. At least three of the six enterprises should be participating in the new health insurance scheme, if applicable.
4 Of the four collective enterprises selected, half should be participating in the new health insurance scheme. It was also thought desirable to include profitable, non-profitable and loss-making enterprises in the sample.

5   Of the four other enterprises included, one should be joint-venture, one joint-stock, one foreign-investment and one privately owned. One or two of the enterprises should be covered by the new scheme, where this had been implemented.

A list of enterprises was compiled, along with information on their respective attributes and economic status. These data were then used to classify them based on the above criteria. Twice the number of enterprises required was then sampled from each category to allow for the possibility that some work units might refuse cooperation.

All the potential enterprises were contacted. A final list of sample work units was then compiled, based on the willingness of the enterprise managers to cooperate with the research team.

A list of all employees was obtained from each work unit and 50 employees were then chosen from this list using systematic sampling. The households of the selected employees were included in the survey and interviews held, initially at the workplace and then at the residence, with the head and key members.

Community-based survey   A sample of 500 households was selected for the community-based survey in each city. These were distributed across the four identified sub-populations (laid-off/unemployed, elderly, registered indigent and migrant), with 200 migrant households sampled and 100 households from each of the other vulnerable groups. Street committees assisted in the identification of the four types of household in the districts selected for the survey. The following detailed criteria were adopted:

•   *Households with laid-off or unemployed worker(s).* Laid-off and unemployed households were defined as those with at least one laid-off or unemployed member who was the main source of family income. Laid-off workers were those who no longer went to work, perhaps temporarily, but who still had some relationship with their former work unit. For example, the worker may have received payment from the employer's insurance fund, or the employer may continue to pay into a pension fund. Unemployed people were those who had lost jobs or never had a job, and who received payments from the Employment Insurance Fund. Both laid-off and unemployed workers are administered by the Labour and Social Security Bureau. A list of names of people who fall into these categories is also kept by the street administrative committees with which they are affiliated. Both sources were used to compile lists from which households were selected using systematic sampling.
•   *Households with elderly people.* These were defined as households with one or more persons over 60 years old and with no children in residence. They could be either retired workers with a pension or people who had never been employed. All were systematically sampled from the lists provided by the street administrative committees.
•   *Poor households.* Mainly those whose income level was below a minimum standard defined by the municipal government, who were identified as poor by

local authorities and received payments from them regularly or occasionally. However, this category also included households which were not officially identified, but were considered extremely poor by the street administrative committees.

• *Migrant households.* A migrant household was defined as one in which all members of the household originated from outside the study cities. They had to have been resident in the city for six months or longer. The households selected were typically those with a husband, wife and children. Single-parent households were also included in the sample, where these consisted of a mother and her children.

Data collection

Different methods of data collection were employed in the work unit- and community-based surveys.

Two rounds of interviews were held with households selected in the work unit-based survey. The first round was undertaken at the work unit. Employees of sampled households were asked to provide basic information about their household and also a home address, telephone number and convenient date for a second interview. They were given a health diary to record information on illness and health care seeking behaviour for each household member over a two-week period.

The second round was undertaken two weeks later. This follow-up interview was intended to gather completed questionnaires from each family member, collect the diary and check responses. The place for the second visit was originally designed to be the employee's home. However, many difficulties arose in attempting to visit all the families selected and it was decided to interview employees at the workplace if they met certain criteria. These criteria included: the employee was an adult woman and clearly aware of what happened to each member of her household over the two-week period, especially the need for and use of health services; the employee was one of the key family members, especially in terms of decision-making at the household level; and no member of the household had given birth in the previous two years, with the exception of the employee. If employees did not meet the criteria, a visit to their home, or at least a telephone interview with other household informants, was required.

In the community-based survey, all the households selected were initially visited by researchers who arranged for interviews to take place in their homes. The interviewers located households according to the addresses provided by the street administrative committees. If no one was at home, the researcher returned again later. If three attempts to visit a household failed, a replacement was substituted.

Pilot study

In order to test the questionnaires and enumeration procedures, a pilot study was carried out in Nantong in August 1999. All the instruments were tested on 100 selected households of which 30 were sampled using the approach described for the community-based study and 70 (in seven work units) using that for the work unit study. All households recorded the health diary.

Fifteen researchers were trained, including five from Shanghai and Shandong universities and ten from the Health Bureau and the Centre of Health Insurance Fund Administration. They participated in the pilot studies on both the household health surveys and the enterprise surveys, and later became the field supervisors in the major data collection phase.

Upon completion of the pilot study, a workshop was held in Shanghai to summarize the results and findings, revise the instruments and finalize the survey procedures and sampling methods.

Selection and training of interviewers
A total of 40 interviewers were chosen from each city for data collection. In Nantong, all the interviewers, besides those participating in the pilot study, were selected from primary health facilities. All the interviewers had some survey experience. In Zibo, 10 people were from Shandong University and 30 were selected from the graduate students of the local medical college or trainees at the Zibo Health School.

A two-day training course was organized in each city. As one component of this training, participants were divided into small groups to conduct at least two interviews. They then discussed with key researchers the problems they had met and the mistakes they had made. All interviewers were examined at the end of the course to test their understanding of the questionnaires.

Quality control
During data collection, a system of quality control was developed to ensure that the data collected were reliable and valid. The interviewers were divided into five groups, consisting of eight people each. Of the eight, one was a key researcher from either Fudan University or Shandong University and acted as the field supervisor responsible for quality control. In addition, there was a group leader who was usually from a local institution and responsible for communication and the organization of daily activities. The remaining six people were divided into three sub-groups.

The first tier of quality control was undertaken at the sub-group level, with each member instructed to check the other's work. The second tier was performed by key researchers from either university. They had to check all the questionnaires completed by three sub-groups and, if anything was found to be wrong or questionable, were required to return the questionnaire to the interviewer for revision. Finally, all completed questionnaires were reviewed by the supervisor. He or she was responsible for checking all the questionnaires and organizing a daily debriefing meeting to provide feedback.

After completing all household interviews, the research team queried some of the information provided. This occurred mainly when the interviewers had been unable to make a second visit to the employee's home, and focused on the possibility that the employee might have missed out information relating to other household members. Telephone calls were made to these households to check and confirm all questionable items. The total number of questionnaires in Nantong to which this problem applied was about 15 per cent of the sample. A further 15 per cent of households were randomly sampled for a telephone confirmation of selected key items. Results of these two types of telephone check are shown in Table A.1.

Table A.1 Results of the two types of telephone quality check*

Type of call	Items checked				
	Total	No. of revisions required	Revision related to health insurance	Revision related to health problems and service use/expense	Others
Calls to households where information was suspect	100	40	18	40	2
Calls to the average household	88	78	8	2	0

* Data in the table do not include those without a telephone or with no response.

From Table A.1, we can see that the quality of the information collected from households meeting the criteria described above was high and the criteria for requiring an interview at an employee's home were appropriate.

Data entry and cleaning
Data coding for the household surveys was conducted before the data were entered into the computer. Epi Info 6.04C was then used to create databases and develop a logic check program for the data entered. Experienced staff and undergraduate students from Shanghai were responsible for data entry. All the data were entered into the computer twice, and then validation was performed to check and correct mistakes. All the databases were validated and cleaned repeatedly until no further errors could be detected.

All questionnaires for the enterprise survey were entered directly into an SPSS (Statistical Package for the Social Sciences) data set. Due to the small number of enterprises involved, data entry and cleaning were relatively straightforward.

Results of the survey
Data on an overall sample of 3,083 households were collected in the two cities: 1,539 in Nantong and 1,544 in Zibo. Details are shown in Tables A.2 and A.3.

The number of valid samples of different categories of household is a little larger than the planned sample size, with the exception of employees in Nantong.

Table A.2 Number of valid households and members: community sample

	Nantong				Zibo			
	Households		Members		Households		Members	
	Number	%	Number	%	Number	%	Number	%
Laid-off	110	19.9	356	25.2	124	23.7	388	27.6
Elderly	119	21.5	246	17.4	103	19.7	224	15.9
Poverty	113	20.4	238	16.9	98	18.7	277	19.7
Migrant	212	38.3	571	40.5	198	37.9	519	36.9
Total	554	100.0	1,411	100.0	523	100.0	1,408	100.0

Table A.3 Number of valid households and members: work unit sample

Work unit category	Nantong				Zibo			
	Households		Members		Households		Members	
	Number	%	Number	%	Number	%	Number	%
1	101	10.3	303	9.6	102	10.0	281	9.5
2	197	20.0	617	19.5	198	19.4	571	19.2
3	293	29.7	924	29.2	319	31.2	928	31.2
4	195	19.8	635	20.1	215	21.1	663	22.3
5	199	20.2	686	21.7	187	18.3	528	17.8
Total	985	100.0	3,165	100.0	1,021	100.0	2,971	100.0

Work Unit Survey

In addition to the household surveys conducted in the two study cities, the project also collected data relating to the selected work units. These included basic information on organization, income level of employees, fiscal status, expenditure on medical care and health insurance. As indicated above, the original intention had been to sample 20 work units in the two cities. However, in Nantong the number of staff in government agencies is small and it was difficult to find one with 50 employees. Therefore two agencies were sampled. One unit in Zibo failed to provide information. Thus data on 21 work units in Nantong and 19 in Zibo were obtained.

A half-day workshop was organized to explain clearly all the required items to the individual nominated by the selected work unit. If any problems were subsequently found, this individual was asked to revise the responses accordingly. The data were initially entered into SPSS, and then transferred to a spreadsheet and analysed using Excel software.

Every work unit was also requested to provide a copy of any available documents outlining their health insurance scheme.

Qualitative Studies on Vulnerable Groups

Key informant interviews

To obtain additional data on vulnerable groups (for example, the size and composition of this population, and government regulations or policies on their access to health and other welfare services) the research team organized a number of key informant interviews. When they conducted these interviews, the researchers also collected relevant documents and information.

The following people from each study city were interviewed by senior researchers from Shanghai:

- The Deputy Director of the Municipal Health Bureau. Questions centred around health service delivery and quality in the context of health sector reform, and focused particularly on the impact of medical insurance on access to health care, especially with regard to the urban poor who had been laid off and lost jobs.
- The Director of the Municipal Civil Affairs Bureau. The interviewers sought to obtain information on the number of disabled people and their entitlements, and access to employment and health services and other welfare services.
- The Deputy Director of the Municipal Labour and Social Security Bureau. The discussion focused on the following: social benefits to which laid-off and unemployed workers are entitled; social security system development, with special reference to medical insurance; income support and re-employment; and loss-making enterprises' participation in medical insurance schemes.
- Managers from two enterprises (one profitable and the other loss-making) were interviewed to understand the issues related to service coverage of medical care through medical or labour insurance schemes, cost of medical care for the enterprises, and impact of medical insurance reform on service use, etc.
- Two hospital managers from each city were also interviewed. The interviews covered the issues of efficiency in service provision, rapid increase of medical care costs and access of the poor to basic health care.

Focus group discussions

Two focus group discussions with health professionals were organized in hospitals in each city. The participants of the discussions represented different health professions working at the hospitals (doctors, nurses, pharmacists, other technicians, etc.). Issues covered included the impact of medical insurance reform on service use and provision, major health problems, changes in efficiency and cost of service provision over the past decade.

Six representatives of the workers' union from five selected enterprises and public institutions in Nantong were invited to attend a focus group discussion on access to, use of, and expenditure on health services among the workers and retirees of these institutions.

One focus group discussion with community (street committee) cadres from the Hongqiao District of Nantong (who participated in the community-based household health survey) was also organized. Topics raised included access of vulnerable people to health care, the medical financial assistance available from the community and government, family planning (with special reference to migrants) and the social security system.

In addition, a focus group discussion with cadres from the Street Administrative Committee, Hongqiao District, Nantong was organized to obtain some insights as to the most vulnerable groups in the city and the social benefits and subsidies they receive from government.

In-depth interviews
About 30 in-depth interviews were conducted with people from five vulnerable groups – the elderly, the poor, laid-off/unemployed workers, migrants and disabled people. Definitions of the first four vulnerable groups have been provided above. The fifth group, disabled people, was defined as those who lacked the abilities of speaking, hearing or seeing, who had lost a limb, or who had mental retardation or long-term mental illness.

Selection of the interviewees In the two study cities, six people from each of the five vulnerable groups were selected for interview. Six elderly people were randomly selected from the households with elderly people included in the community-based household survey. The same approach was used to select the poor, laid off/unemployed and migrant households. Six disabled persons were selected using the list of disabled people provided by several street administrative committees. These had been compiled according to the regulations and policies on disability developed by the municipal Civil Affairs Bureau. Figure A.1 illustrates how these individuals were chosen from the different vulnerable groups for the in-depth interviews.

Organization of the in-depth interviews Experienced senior researchers from Shanghai and Shandong took the major responsibility for the in-depth interviews. Three people from Nantong Medical Insurance Administration Centre and the Municipal Health Bureau were also recruited to conduct interviews after they had received proper training. All the interviews were held at the interviewee's home and all were tape-recorded. An assistant from the research team participated in the interviews and took notes throughout. Usually the head of the household or a key member were the main respondents. During the process of the interviews, the interviewers were asked to observe the interviewee's expression, emotion and living environment, and to record these findings in the notes. Upon completion of the interview, a small gift was given to the household as a token of appreciation.

All the interviews used semi-structured questionnaires. In order to ensure that these questionnaires were appropriate, a pilot study was performed to test the instrument before the exercise. In this pilot study, the team selected for interview one individual from each of five vulnerable groups in Nantong.

Analysis of the qualitative data collected Transcripts of each interview were prepared from the tape recording. The researchers checked these transcripts with the notes taken during the interviews. Once the transcripts were finalized, analysis of the information was performed based on both the initial research questions and the themes arising during the study.

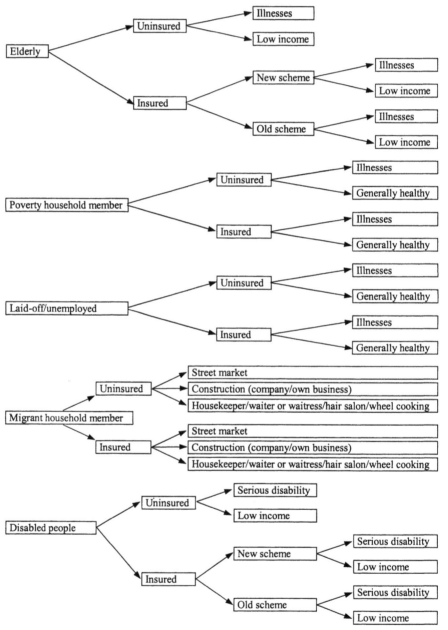

Figure A.1 Diagram demonstrating the selection of people from vulnerable groups for in-depth interview

Hospital Efficiency Study

This section presents the methods employed in the hospital efficiency study conducted in Nantong and Zibo. It is divided into five sub-sections covering: the purpose of the study; the conceptual (theoretical) framework; data sources, sampling size and sampling technique; descriptive and statistical analysis; and problems and adjustment of methodology.

Purpose

The objectives of the efficiency study were to examine the association between health care reform and changes in facility management, and to explore the outcome in terms of the implications for efficiency. The changes in facility management relate to both external and internal factors. The external factors include changes in sources of finance, composition of facility income and pricing of health services. The way in which hospitals receive their revenues has also to be considered. Various payment methods are practiced including fee-for-service, fixed charge, capitation and diagnosis related groups (DRGs).

It was intended to analyse the detailed contractual mechanisms between the provider and the different payers. Given those external factors that constrain hospital behaviour, there is still scope for internal monitoring and management of resources which providers decide on themselves (though they may also be regulated by government rules). The internal monitoring systems relate to internal budgeting, fund retention to regulate performance and methods used to reward facility employees (bonus, etc.). It is also of interest to analyse how hospitals have used their autonomy with regard to investment in construction and equipment technologies. Special attention has been paid to the procedures governing the use of drugs and other medicinal materials.

Finally the relationship between health care reforms/facility management and efficiency of the hospital sector has been examined. This has been done by presenting descriptive performance indicators, such as unit cost analysis and utilization measures. Productivity analysis has been carried out based on the method of data envelopment analysis (DEA). All output measures have also been adjusted for quality and case mix. An explanatory model has been created to explain the differences in productivity across the hospitals.

Conceptual Framework

The study is concerned with the relationship between changes in the hospitals' environment, particularly those relating to health care reforms, and the impact on hospital behaviour and efficiency. Given that Chinese hospitals have been given a considerable degree of autonomy, the study attempts to find out how this freedom has been used and what restrictions they are facing. It seeks to measure and explain the efficiency of the hospital sector by relating the performance to health care reform changes. The first part is a pure efficiency study wherein different analyses are used to relate the use of inputs to produced outputs. Descriptive efficiency measures and unit cost measures are used for all hospitals and a number of departments within the hospitals.

The second part tries to explain behaviour by relating the hospital performance to the changes in the environment. It attempts to uncover which types of internal monitoring mechanisms have been developed and used by hospitals. Figure A.2 provides the general framework for analysis.

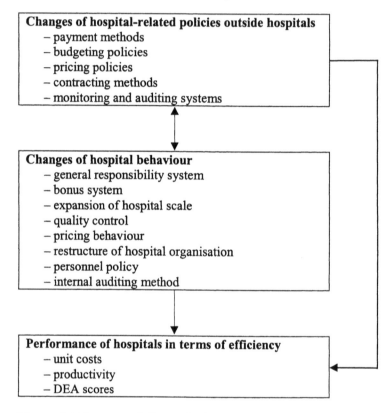

Figure A.2 Framework for exploring the relations between changes to hospital environments and behaviour, and changes in hospital efficiency

In assessing the likely impact of changes to payment systems and contractual relationships, it is important to bear in mind that the underlying nature of demand from patients is unchanged and that patients with insurance coverage are not very sensitive to user charges. It is most likely that this and the increased autonomy of providers in a competitive market will result in non-price competition. The role of keeping costs down will rest on different third party payers (government and/or health insurance schemes) who will be in the best position to exert cost containment.

Data Sources and Sampling Procedure

The data sources are varied and are both quantitative and qualitative in nature. In order to analyse efficiency as well as try to explain the changes, several sources were used which are summarized below:

- Hospital survey for data on expenditures, staff, equipment, performance and structure of hospitals for the period 1985 to 1999. The sample consisted of 22 hospitals in Zibo and 19 hospitals in Nantong. In each hospital specific data were collected from departmental level for major clinics;
- Official documents from the hospitals and health authorities;
- Key informant interviews and focus group discussions with hospital managers and representatives from health authorities;
- A tracer condition study.

Hospital survey

As the focus of the study is on the hospital sector, a sampling strategy was used to include the most common types of Chinese hospitals. The sample consisted exclusively of hospitals from two levels: municipal and county. Smaller hospitals with few beds, so-called township hospitals, were excluded. There were no tertiary/university hospitals in the two study cities. With this sampling strategy all hospitals at municipal and county levels were included (22 in Zibo and 19 in Nantong). The hospitals were also categorized into different types (general hospitals, Chinese hospitals and enterprise hospitals).

A questionnaire was developed covering specific items: hospital background data; sources and size of revenues; categories of expenditure; use of inputs and equipment; and performance in terms of outputs and quality outcomes. Most questions referred to the whole hospital, but some were specifically about hospital departments. The indicators in the hospital study included: unit costs and case mix (financial documents, facility questionnaire and stratified samples of financial and medical records), and quality of care (stratified samples of medical records and current patients).

The questionnaire was managed and filled in by the investigators who met representatives from the hospitals (departments of finance, accounting, etc.). The questionnaire was completed with the assistance of the hospital representatives and was based on reviews of financial and medical documents and records. Discussions were held about unclear information and a second interview was made if necessary if data were missing or invalid.

Official documents from hospitals and health authorities

The purpose of collecting documents was to get background information about the health care reforms that had affected the hospitals, and to find out how these had influenced hospital policy and management. An additional aim was to obtain information about changes of internal facility management. Specific information was collected to understand the implementation and structure of the staff bonus/reward system, personnel policies and the responsibility system. Existing data including health policy documents and statistical information were collected by consulting relevant health officials and reviewing related statistical books and reports. The investigators visited each hospital to collect the documents.

This information was then used to create 'dummy variables' (yes/no) which were later used in the explanatory analysis of efficiency. In addition to documents from the hospitals, similar information on the topic of health care reforms was collected from the local health authorities. Particular attention was paid to issues about health insurance, price regulations and payment methods to hospitals.

Key informant interviews and focus group discussion
A survey of key informant interviews and focus group discussions was conducted in each city using open and semi-structured questions. The interviewees were hospital managers and representatives from the health authorities. Health workers and patients were also interviewed. The overall question raised in connection with various aspects was the impact of health policy on the performance of hospitals in terms of management, efficiency and costs of services.

The tracer study
The tracer study was based on a medical record review in which two health conditions, acute appendicitis and normal birth delivery, were targeted. Medical records of 888 patients with acute appendicitis and 891 patients who had given birth from three Zibo hospitals in 1995 and 1999 were surveyed. The purpose of tracing the medical records was to examine differences in medical expenses under different health insurance plans with different payment methods. Indicators used included patients' personal information (age, sex, occupation), health insurance coverage, medical procedures received (diagnosis and procedure), categorized items of medical expenses and payment methods.

Descriptive and Statistical Analysis

The initial step taken in the analysis was to adjust the performance data for differences in case mix and quality. Differences in case mix in particular might lead to unfair comparison of performance for hospitals admitting severe cases.

Adjustment of case mix
Severity of illness has a close relation with medical expenses. Patients with severe conditions cost more than others. The adjustment of case mix for in-patient services was based on the diagnosis. A case mix index (CMI) that is widely used for such adjustment was employed. The formula to calculate CMI is as follows.

$$CMI_j = \frac{\sum(C_jX * P_jX)}{\sum(CX * PX)}$$

Where CMI_j is the value of CMI of j hospital, C_jX is the average expense of j hospital, CX is the standard expense of X disease, P_j is the proportion of patients with X disease in j hospital, and PX is the proportion of patients with X diseases in total patients of sample hospitals. By considering the differences in the share of patients with different diseases the total output could be weighted. For out-patient services there is a lack of diagnosis data. In the study, the average expense per out-patient service was used to adjust the case mix of out-patient services. In order to avoid unstable expenses across years, the medical expenses of each hospital in the four selected years were averaged.

Adjustment of quality
Comparison of relative service efficiency levels of different hospitals requires that quality of care should be adjusted to be equal across the hospitals. In this study, a quality adjusted index (QAI) was used to adjust the quality of sample hospitals. The formula for calculating QAI is:

$$QAI = X = \sum_{i=1}^{n} X_i/S_i * W_i \qquad (1)$$

Where X_i are the factual numbers of indicators, S_i are the standard numbers of indicators, and W_i are the weights representing importance of selected indicators in determining quality. X_i were obtained from the survey, S_i were set by the Ministry of Health, and W_i were provided by medical experts. From 50 indicators that are usually used for assessing quality of hospital services, six were selected by a panel of medical experts. Selected indicators include recovery rates of hospitalized patients, consistent rates of diagnosis before and after discharge of in-patients, consistent rates of diagnosis before and after physical operations, rates of successfully rescuing emergency cases, rates of qualified nursing, and hospital infectious rates. Those indicators represent key procedures of diagnosis, treatment and nursing in out-patient, in-patient and surgical care facilities. Table A.4 shows the variables for measuring QAI.

Table A.4 Indicators used for calculating the quality adjusted index

Indicators	S_i (%)	Weights
Recovery rates of hospitalized patients	≥93.7	0.190
Consistent rates of diagnosis before and after discharges	≥95.0	0.172
Consistent rates of diagnosis before and after physical operations	≥90.0	0.170
Rates of successfully rescuing emergency cases	≥80.0	0.185
Rates of qualified nursing work	≥90.0	0.172
Hospital internal infectious rates	≤10.0	0.126

The figures above for each hospital were substituted into formula (1). Values of QAI of each hospital in 1999 were obtained as listed above. There are no considerable variations in values of QAI among the hospitals. Values of QAI in

1990, 1995, and 1997 were also calculated. Those values are used in the productivity calculation.

Descriptive statistics and unit costs analysis
In the first part of the analysis some background variables for total revenues and expenditure were compared with similar data for China and Shandong and Jiangsu Provinces. All revenue and expenditure data were calculated in fixed prices in order to compare figures over time. Hospital expenditure and utilization trends were compared in order to gauge how representative were the data collected from the two cities. Descriptive data of the hospital expenditure and utilization were collected for different types of hospitals. The unit costs analysis was performed by calculation of the following measures:

- Out-patient services per doctor;
- Bed-days per doctor;
- Revenues per health worker;
- Occupancy rate for in-patient care;
- Average length of stay;
- Turnover days;
- Cost per out-patient visit;
- Cost per in-patient admission.

For all these indicators an adjustment has been made for quality and case mix. For comparison over time all costs were calculated in fixed prices. In addition to the measures above, several other output measures, such as emergency cases, discharged patients and surgical operations, were analysed.

Productivity analysis and models for determining efficiency
A problem with unit cost analysis and other descriptive measures of efficiency is how to incorporate and put a weight on several outputs delivered by hospitals. An analysis of the multidimensional activities in which hospitals are engaged requires methods for concentrating outputs into a single number reflecting performance. DEA is used to estimate the efficiency of the hospitals sector. The method is a non-parametric technique which uses linear programming to measure the magnitude of departure from efficiency frontiers for each decision-making unit (e.g. a hospital) based on their use of resources to produce multiple outputs. To put it simply, the DEA is basically a benchmarking practice where the most efficient units form an efficient frontier to which all other units' performance is related.

DEA is a convenient method for several reasons. First, it can handle multiple-output activities. The method does not require the input or the cost side to be expressed in monetary terms. It can use information about inputs such as number of staff and number of beds instead. Hence, factoring prices for each input is not a necessary requirement. The DEA method allows for a certain number of total inputs and outputs depending on the size of the sample. As a rule of thumb the sample size (n) should exceed the sum of all inputs and outputs by several times.

Hence, different models have been tested where different combinations of inputs and outputs have been used.

In order to explain the changes of hospital behaviour and related performance several explanatory models have been set up. In these models different hypothesis have been formulated regarding which factors (external and internal) influence the behaviour of hospitals. These explanations could be summarized in the following categories:

- Ownership, administrative relations, type of hospital;
- Sources and mix of finance, payment system (external reimbursement);
- Bonus system (year of turning point of methods) and design of general responsibility system (internal incentives and monitoring systems);
- Personnel policy;
- Changes in hospital scales: increase rates of capital input (personnel, beds);
- The dependence of sales of drugs;
- Structure of hospitals and use of high-technology equipment.

The explanatory models are analysed by using multiple regression analysis where the significant explanatory variables are discussed. Several models are used for different measures of DEA and other performance variables. The basic model can be shown by Figure A.3.

Problems and Adjustment of Methodology

There were a number of methodology-related problems (for example, adjustment) which explains why the study somewhat deviates from the original proposal. As there was a limitation on the sample size and the scope of the study was to focus on the hospital sector and hospital efficiency, a choice had to be made concerning which categories of hospital to concentrate on. In addition, the study looked at efficiency of urban health reforms, and in the urban areas the hospitals at municipal and county level supply most of specialized care. Hence, it was decided to exclude the community health centres or township hospitals from the sample.

There was also a lack of medical information on disease categories and diagnosis for out-patient care, which resulted in some assumptions being made when calculating case mix for out-patient care. Also the quality indicators had to rely on existing information.

Another circumstance which lay outside the influence of the research team was the late implementation of the new health insurance reform in the city of Zibo. This made it impossible to make a before and after study of the impact of the reform. Still, the situation gave the team an interesting comparison between Zibo and the city of Nantong where the reform had been implemented.

Independent variables   Dependent variables

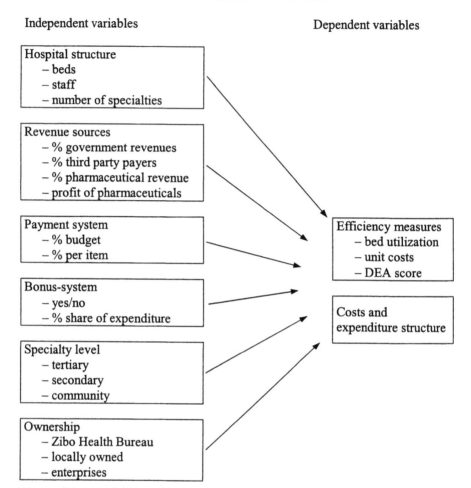

Figure A.3 A model for explaining hospitals' efficiency performance

Bibliography

Adler, P.A. and Adler, P. (1994), 'Observational Techniques', in N. Denzin and Y.S. Lincoln, (eds), *Handbook of Qualitative Research*, Sage, London, pp. 377–93.

All China Women's Federation Research Institute (1991), *Statistics on Chinese Women 1949–1989*, China Statistical Publishing House, Beijing.

Asian Development Bank (1999), *Policy for the Health Sector*, Asian Development Bank, Manila, pp. 5–14.

Barer, M. *et al*. (1987), 'Ageing and Health Care Utilization: New Evidence on Old Fallacies', *Social Science and Medicine*, Vol. 24(10), pp. 851–62.

Bloom, G. (2001), 'Equity in Health in Unequal Societies: Meeting Health Needs in Contexts of Social Change', *Health Policy*, Vol. 57(3), pp. 205–24.

Bloom, G. and Fang, J. (2003), 'China's Rural Health System in a Changing Institutional Context', *IDS Working Paper*, No. 194, Institute of Development Studies, Brighton.

Bloom, G., Han, L. and Li, X. (2000), 'How Health Workers Earn a Living in China', *IDS Working Paper*, No. 108, Institute of Development Studies, Brighton.

Cai, R. (1999), 'Pilot Study on Urban Health Insurance Reform in Zhenjiang. Report on Health Financing Studies', National Institute of Health Economics, Beijing.

Cai, R.H. (2001), 'Review of the Basic Medical Insurance System Reform in Urban China', paper presented at the National Workshop on Reforming Health Services for Equity and Efficiency in Urban China, Beijing, 4–6 December 2001.

Cai, W. (2000), 'How is Urban Health Insurance Reform Correctly Assessed?' *Health Economics Research*, Vol. 43, pp. 34–6.

CASS (Chinese Academy of Social Sciences) (1998), Project Group on Social Development in China, 'Institutional Reforms and Challenges at the Middle Stage of China's Reform', *Social Sciences in China*, Vol. 19(2), pp. 83–93.

CASS (Chinese Academy of Social Sciences) (2000), Research Group on China's Social Security System, 'A Study of China's Social Security System', *Social Sciences in China*, Vol. 21(4), pp. 50–59.

Centre for Health Statistics and Information (1998), *National Health Services Survey Report*, Ministry of Health, Beijing.

Chan, Wingchan and Zhang, Li (1999), 'The Hukou System and Rural-Urban Migration', *China Quarterly*, p. 618.

Chen, C. and Wang, Y. (2000), 'Discussing the Nutrition and Economical Development in Poor Area', *Health Research*, Vol. 29(5), pp. 305–7.

Chen, J. and Wang, G. (2000), 'Analysis of Health Services Utilization and Its Influencing Factors of Limb Handicapped People in Urban Tangshan', *Modern Preventive Medicine*, Vol. 27(2), pp. 193–5.

Chen, J.X., Xu, K.Q., Chen, J.X. and Qing, M.Z. (1998), 'The Infectious Diseases Trend in Nantong During 1956–95', *Jiang Shu Preventive Medicine*, Vol. 1, pp. 39–40.

Chen, M.J., Li, Y., Wang, H. *et al*. (1999), 'Analysis of Medical Cost and its Structure for an Inpatient Admittance in General Hospital', *Chinese Health Services Management*, Vol. 18(11), pp. 287–9.

Chen, Q.Z. and Guo, W.B. (2000), 'A Survey of Psychological Health of Laid-off Workers', *Journal of Health Psychology*, Vol. 8(4), pp. 465–8.

Chen, X. (2000), 'Health Problems and Countermeasures During Urbanisation', *Medicine and Society*, Vol. 13(3), pp. 1–3.

China Health Statistical Abstract (1998), National Health Statistical Centre, Beijing.

China Labour Statistic Yearbook (1998), China Statistical Publishing House, Beijing.

China Labour Statistic Yearbook (2000), China Statistical Publishing House, Beijing.

China Rights Forum (1998), 'Report on Implementation of CEDAW in the People's Republic of China', December 1998, www.hrichina.org/download_repository/A/cedaw%2098.doc (accessed February 2004).

China Social Insurance (1998), 'Memorandum of Health Insurance Reform: Trace of Vicissitudes of Health Insurance System for Employees', *China Social Insurance*, Vol. 7, pp. 9–11.

China State Council (2000), *Decision About the Urban Health Insurance Reform*, Economics Press, Beijing.

China Statistical Yearbook (2000), China Statistical Publishing House, Beijing.

China Statistical Yearbook (2001), China Statistical Publishing House, Beijing.

Chinese Communist Party Committee and State Council (1997), *Decision on Developing and Reforming Health Care System*, Beijing.

Cook, S., 2001, 'After the Iron Rice Bowl: Extending the Safety Net in China', *IDS Discussion Paper*, No. 377, Institute of Development Studies, Brighton.

Cook, S. and Jolly, S. (2001), 'Unemployment, Poverty and Gender in Urban China: Perceptions and Experiences of Laid-off Workers in Three Chinese Cities', *IDS Research Report*, No. 50, Institute of Development Studies, Brighton.

Cook, S. and White, G. (1998), 'Changing Pattern of Poverty in China: Issues for Research and Policy', *IDS Working Paper*, No. 67, Institute of Development Studies, Brighton.

Croll, E. (1999), 'Social Welfare Reforms: Trends and Tensions', *China Quarterly*, No. 50, pp. 684–99.

Das Gupta, M., Lee, S., Uberoi, P., Wang, D., Wang, L. and Zang, X. (2000), 'State Policies and Women's Autonomy in China, The Republic of Korea, and India 1950–2000: Lessons from Contrasting Experiences', Policy Research Report on Gender and Development Working Paper Series, No. 16, World Bank, available at www.worldbank.org/gender/prr (accessed 2 February 2004).

Davin, D. (1990), 'Chinese Models of Development and Their Implications for Women', in I. Tinker (ed.), *Persistent Inequalities, Women and World Development*, Oxford University Press, Oxford.

Deng P., Mi, G.M., Wang Y.C. *et al.* (1999), 'Study of Health Services Demand of Elderly People in an Urban Community', *Chinese General Practice*, Vol. 3(5), pp. 373–4.

Denzin, N.K. (1994), 'The Art and Politics of Interpretation', in N. Denzin and Y.S. Lincoln (eds), *Handbook of Qualitative Research*, Sage, London, pp. 500–515.

Dong, W. (2003), 'Healthcare-financing Reforms in Transitional Society: A Shanghai Experience', *Journal of Health and Population Research*, Vol. 21(3), pp. 223–34.

Dranove, D. (1998), 'Pricing by Non-profit Institution: The Case of Hospital Cost-shifting', *Journal of Health Economics*, Vol. 7, pp. 47–57.

Druschel, K. (1999), 'Urban Working Women and Constructions of Gender Equality in the People's Republic of China', thesis presented for A.B. degree with honours in International Relations, Kenyon College, Gambier, Ohio.

Du, Lexun, Ma, Jin, Ju, Xiuron *et al.* (1998), 'Time Series Analysis of Health Account', *Chinese Journal of Health Resources*, Vol. 1, pp. 3–6.

Ensor, T. (1999), 'Developing Health Insurance in Transitional Asia', *Social Science and Medicine*, Vol. 48, pp. 871–9.

Fan, Q. (1989), *Compendium of Literature on Price and Price Reform in China*, Development Economics Research Programme, CP No. 2, London School of Economics, London.

Feng, X. (1997), 'The Costs and Benefits of Rural-Urban Migration', *Social Sciences in China*, Vol. 18(4), pp. 52–65.

Feng, Y. (1999), 'Social Security and Economic Development: Lessons From Other Countries and Emergence of a Modern Social Security System in China – An Introduction', *International Journal of Economic Development*, Vol. 1(4).

Flick, U. (1992), 'Triangulation Revisited: Strategy of or Alternative to Validation of Qualitative Data', *Journal for the Theory of Social Behavior*, Vol. 22, pp. 175–97.

Fu, L. (1953), 'Our Journal', *Chinese Medical Journal*, Vol. 69(1), pp. 1–2.

Gansu Provincial Department of Health (2000), 'History and Development of Health Care System in Gansu', unpublished data, Gansu.

Gao, J. and Tang, S. (2000), 'Health Insurance and Hospitalisation in Urban China: Bending to the Wind of Change', *World Hospitals and Health Services*, Vol. 36(3).

Gao, J., Tang S., Tolhurst, R. and Rao, K. (2001), 'Changing Access to Health Services in Urban China: Implications For Equity?', *Health Policy and Planning*, Vol. 16(3), pp. 302–12.

Gao, Jinhua (2000), 'Chengshi dibao: fugaimian zhubu kuoda, guanli gengjia guifan' [Urban Minimum Living Security: Gradually Expanding Coverage and Standardising Management], *Zhongguo Minzheng [China Civil Affairs]*.

Gong, H. (2001), 'Present Three Most Concerning Issues to the General Public', Beijing: *Zhongguo Guoqing Guoli*, No. 5 (cited in Dong, 2003).

Goodkind, D. and West, L. (2002), 'China's Floating Population: Definitions, Data and Recent Findings', *Urban Studies*, Vol. 39(12), pp. 2237–50.

Gu, E. (2003), 'Labour Market Insecurities in China', www.ilo.org/public/english/ protection/ses/download/docs/labour_china.pdf (accessed 28 July 2003).

Gu, X. and Tang, S. (1995), 'Reform of the Chinese Health Care Financing Systems', *Health Policy*, Vol. 32, pp. 1–3. Also in P. Berman (ed.), *Health Sector Reform in Developing Countries – Making Health Development Sustainable*, Harvard University Press, Cambridge.

Guan, Xinping (1999), 'Zhongguo chengshi pinkun wenti yanjiu' [Research on China's Urban Poverty Problem], *Hunan Renmin Chubanshe*.

Gustafsson, B. and Li, S. (2000), 'Economic Transformation and the Gender Earnings Gap in Urban China', *Journal of Population Economics*, Vol. 13, pp. 305–29.

Hadley, J. and Feder, J. (1985), 'Hospital Cost-shifting and Care for the Uninsured', *Health Affairs*, Vol. 4, pp. 67–80.

Han, L. and Zhang, Z. (1999), 'Medicaid for Poverty', *Chinese Health Economics*, Vol. 18(11), pp. 25–32.

Hao, M., Luo, L., Jiang, X.P. *et al.* (1999), 'A Synopsis of a Series of Studies on Community Health Services', *Chinese Journal of Hospital Administration*, Vol. 15(8).

Hao, M. and Xu, G.R. (1994), 'Comparative Analysis on the Features of Health Development in Poor and Rich Districts', *Chinese Primary Health Care*, Vol. 8(4), pp. 3–6.

Hartmann, B. (1995), *Reproductive Rights and Wrongs*, South End Press, Boston.

Hay, J. (1983), 'The Impact of Public Health Care Financing Policies on Private Sector Hospital Costs', *Journal of Health Politics, Policy and Law*, Vol. 7, pp. 945–52.

Horn, J. (1969), *Away With All Pests, An English Surgeon in the People's Republic of China: 1954–1969*, Hamlyn, London.

Howell, J. (1997), 'The Chinese Economic Miracle and Urban Workers', *European Journal of Development Research*, Vol. 9(2), pp. 148–75.

Hu, A. (1999), 'The Biggest Adjustment for Entering the New Century: China Enters a Period of High Unemployment' [Zhongguo, guoqing fenxi yanjiu baogao], CASS and Qinghua University, cited in Cook (2001).

Hu, H. (1996), 'Regulation of Medical High Technologies in China', in *Reforming Health Financing Policy*, Chinese Economics Press, Beijing, pp. 135–42.

Hu, S. and Gong, X. (1999), 'Assessment of Drug Expenditures in China', *Chinese Journal of Health Economics*, Vol. 16, pp. 9–12.

Hu, Tehwei, Ong, M., Lin, Zihua and Li, E. (1999), 'The Effects of Economic Reform on Health Insurance and the Financial Burden for Urban Workers in China', *Health Economics*, Vol. 8, pp. 309–21.

Hu, X. (1996), 'Reducing State-owned Enterprises' Social Burdens and Establishing a Social Insurance System', in H.G. Broadman (ed.), *Policy Options for Reform of Chinese State-Owned Enterprises*, World Bank Discussion Paper, No. 335, World Bank, Washington, D.C., pp. 125–48.

Hu, X. and Gong, X. (1999), 'Appraise the Increase in the Cost of Health Care', *China Health Economics*, Vol. 18(6), pp. 9–12.

Huang, S. and Wang, Y. (1997), 'The Socialization of Health Insurance', *Chinese Primary Health Care*, Vol. 11(2), pp. 14–15.

Huang, W. (1999), 'Study on the Quality of Life of the Elderly in the Urban Area of Guiyang', *Practical Preventive Medicine*, Vol. 6(5), pp. 321–2.

Hussain, A. (1999), 'Social Welfare in China in the Context of Three Transitions', unpublished paper, Asia Research Centre, London School of Economics, London.

Hussain, A. (2000), 'Living in the City', *China Review*, Spring, pp. 8–11.

Hussain, A. (2003), *Urban Poverty in China: Measurement, Patterns and Policies*, InFocus Programme on Socio-Economic Security, International Labour Organization, Geneva.

Jiangsu Provincial Government (1999), *Fee Schedule for Hospitals*, Jiangsu Provincial Government, Nanjing.

Krieg, R. and Schädler, M. (1995), 'Soziale Sicherheit im China der neunziger Jahre', *Mitteilungen des Instituts für Asienkunde,* No. 245, Hamburg.

Leon, D., Walt, G. and Gilson, L. (2001), 'International Perspectives on Health Inequality and Policy', *Journal of British Medicine*, Vol. 322, pp. 591–4.

Leung, J.C.B. (1995), 'The Political Economy of Unemployment and Unemployment Insurance in the People's Republic of China', *International Social Work*, Vol. 38(2), pp. 139–49.

Li, Chunling (2002), 'The Class Structure of China's Urban Society During the Transitional Period', *Social Sciences in China*, Vol. 23(1), pp. 91–9.

Li, Jiewei (1998), 'Impact of Health Insurance Reform on Behaviour of Drug Prescription', *Chinese Hospital Management*, Vol. 6, pp. 23–5.

Li, L. (1999), 'Family Insurance or Social Insurance. Policy Options for China's Social Reform', *International Journal of Economic Development*, Vol. 1(4).

Li, Peilin (2002), 'Changes in Social Stratification in China Since the Reform', *Social Sciences in China*, Vol. 23(1), pp. 42–7.

Li, Y. *et al.* (2000), 'Investigation on Psychological Health Situation of Laid-off People', *Health Psychological Journal*, Vol. 8(1), pp. 80–84.

Liang, H. (1999), 'Key Problems and Reform Recommendations to Health Development in Shanghai Pudong Economic Zone', *Chinese Health Economics*, Vol. 18(5), pp. 18–20.

Lieberthal, K. and Oksenberg, M. (1988), *Policy Making in China – Leaders, Structures, and Processes*, Princeton University Press, Princeton.

Lieverdink, H. (2001), 'The Marginal Success of Regulated Competition Policy in the Netherlands', *Social Sciences and Medicine*, Vol. 52, pp. 1183–94.

Lin, S. (1999), 'The Effect of an Expansion of the Pay-as-You-Go Social Security System in China', *International Journal of Economic Development*, Vol. 1(4).

Liu, G. *et al.* (2002), 'China's Urban Health Insurance Reform Experiment in Zhengjiang: Cost and Utilisation Analysis', in T.W. Hu and C.R. Hsieh (eds), *The Economics of Health Care in Asia-Pacific Countries*, Edward Elgar, Aldershot.

Liu, G., Cai, R., Zhao, Z., Yuen, P., Xiong, X., Chao, S. and Wang, B. (1999), 'Urban Health Care Reform Initiative in China: Findings from 1st Pilot Experiment in Zhengjian City', *International Journal of Economic Development*, Vol. 1(4).

Liu, S. and MacKellar, L. (2001), 'Key Issues of Ageing and Social Security in China', Interim Report IR-01-004/January, International Institute for Applied Systems Analysis, Laxenburg.

Liu, X. (1999), 'Evaluation of Social Health Insurance Reform in China', *International Journal of Economic Development*, Vol. 1(4).

Liu, X and Hsiao, W. (1995), 'The Cost Escalation of Social Health Insurance Plan in China: Its Implication for Public Policy', *Social Sciences and Medicine*, Vol. 41, pp. 1095–101.

Liu, X. and Zhan, S. (2000), 'Health Care for Floating People', *Straits Preventive Medicine*, Vol. 6(1), pp. 17–19.

Liu, Xinming (1991), 'Rationales for Reforming Government Health Insurance Scheme', *Chinese Health Economics*, Vol. 3, pp. 3–4.

Liu, X.Y. (2003), 'Decentralization and its Impact on Health Human Resource Management: A Case Study in Longyan Prefecture, Fujian Province', unpublished PhD thesis, Fudan University, Shanghai.

Liu, Y. (2002), 'Reforming China's Urban Health Insurance System', *Health Policy*, Vol. 60, pp. 133–50.

Liu, Yunguo and Bloom, G. (2002), 'Designing a Rural Health Reform Project: The Negotiation of Change in China', *IDS Working Paper*, No. 150, Institute of Development Studies, Brighton.

Lu, W. *et al.* (2000), 'Exploring the Health Insurance Issue for Laid-off People', *Chinese Health Management*, Vol. 16(2), pp. 87–8.

Luo, Wujing and Hu, Shanlian (1998), 'Socio-economic Development and Health Financing', *Medicine and Philosophy*, Vol. 5, pp. 23–6.

Ma, J. and Zhai, F. (2001), 'Financing China's Pension Reform', presented to the International Conference on China and the WTO: the Financial Challenge, Kennedy School, Harvard University.

Ma, Q. (2000), 'How to Enhance Preventive Health Administration to Floating Workers in Building Sites', *Chinese Health Service Management*, Vol. 19(6), p. 52.

Maurer-Fazio, M., Rawski, T.G. and Zhang, W. (1999), 'Inequality in the Rewards for Holding up Half the Sky: Gender Wage Gaps in China's Urban Labour Market, 1998–1994', *The China Journal*, Vol. 41, pp. 55–88.

Melnick G., Zwanziger, J. and Pattison, P. (1992), 'The Effects of Market Structure and Bargaining Position on Hospital Prices', *Journal of Health Economics*, Vol. 11, pp. 217–33.

Meng, Q., Bian, Y. and Ge, R. (1998), *Report on Costing of Hospitals in China*, Centre for Cost Accounting and Analysis, Ministry of Health, Beijing.

Meng, Q., Bian, Y., Ge, R., Sun, Q. *et al.* (2002), 'Pricing Policy of Health Care: Problems, Causes, and Policy Options', *Chinese Journal of Health Economics*, Vol. 5, pp. 23–5.

Meng, Q., Sun, Q. and Hearst, N. (2002), 'Hospital Charge Exemptions for the Poor in Shandong, China', *Health Policy and Planning*, Vol.17(Suppl. 1), pp. 56–63.

Meng, Q., Zhuang, N., Bian, Y. *et al.* (2001), 'Impact of Urban Health Reform on Hospital Efficiency', in Proceedings of Conference on Reforming Health Services for Equity and Efficiency in Urban China, Beijing, 4–6 December 2001.

Mills, A., Bennett, S., Siriwanarangsun, P. and Tangcharoensathien, V. (2000), 'The Response of Providers to Capitation Payment: A Case Study from Thailand', *Health Policy*, Vol. 51, pp. 163–80.

Milwertz, C.N. (1997), *Accepting Population Control. Urban Chinese Women and the One-Child Family Policy*, Curzon Press, Richmond.

Ministry of Finance and Ministry of Health (1999), *Hospital Accounting Guideline*, Beijing.

Ministry of Health (1989), *Health Statistics Information in China: 1949–1988*, Beijing.

Ministry of Health (1995), *Hospital Accounting Reports*, Beijing.

Ministry of Health (1996), Data on annual national health statistics in China, Beijing.

Ministry of Health (1998a), *Health Resources and Utilisation Since 1980s*, Statistical and Information Centre, Ministry of Health, Beijing.

Ministry of Health (1998b), *Research on National Health Services – An Analysis Report of the Second National Health Services Survey in 1998*, Beijing.

Ministry of Health (1999a), *Research Analysis on National Health Service*, Beijing.

Ministry of Health (1999b), *Report on National Health Services Survey of 1998*, Beijing.

Ministry of Health (2000), *Health Statistical Yearbook*, People's Publishing House of Health, Beijing.

Ministry of Health (2001), *Report on Hospital Financial Accounting*, Beijing.

Ministry of Health (2002), *Abstracts of Health Statistics and Information*, Beijing.

Ministry of Health and Ministry of Education (2000), *Study on Chinese Development of Medical Education*, Beijing.

Nantong Bureau of Statistics (2000), *Nantong Statistical Yearbook*, Nantong.

Nantong Health Insurance Management Centre (2001), 'Introduction of Nantong Health Insurance System Reform', unpublished document, Nantong.

National Bureau of Statistics (2000), *China Statistical Yearbook*, China Statistical Publishing House, Beijing.

National Bureau of Statistics (2001), *China Statistical Yearbook*, China Statistical Publishing House, Beijing.

National Committee of Administrative System Reform of China *et al.* (1996), *Reforming Employees' Medical Security Scheme*, Reform Publishing House, Beijing, pp. 69–215.

Ning, H. *et al.* (1999), 'An Epidemiological Study on Quality of Life among Elderly Population in Shenzhen', *Chinese Journal of Prevention and Control of Chronic Non-communicated Diseases*, Vol. 7(4), pp. 168–70.

Ou, A.H. and Zhu, Y. (2000), 'Analysis of Condition of Elderly People and Their Health Service Utilisation in Guiyang City', *Chinese Primary Health Care*, Vol. 14(3), pp. 47–8.

Oxaal, Z. and Cook, S. (1998), 'Health and Poverty: A Gender Analysis', BRIDGE (Development-Gender) On-line Reports, No. 46, The Institute of Development Studies, Brighton.

Patton, M.Q. (1990), *Qualitative Evaluation and Research Methods*, 2nd edn, Sage, London.

Propper C. (1996), 'Market Structure and Prices: The Responses of Hospitals in the UK National Health Services to Competition', *Journal of Public Economics*, Vol. 61, pp. 307–35.

Qiu, Y. *et al.* (1999), 'Investigation on Child Health Situation in Floating People', *Chinese Primary Health Care*, Vol. 13(5), p. 31.

Rice, T., Stearns, S,. Desharnais, S., Pathman, D. *et al.* (1996), 'Do Physicians Cost Shift?' *Health Affairs*, Vol. 15(3), pp. 215–25.

Rofel, L. (1999), *Other Modernities: Gendered Yearning in China After Socialism*, University of California Press, Berkeley.
Selden, M. and Lou, L. (1997), 'The Reform of Social Welfare in China', *World Development*, Vol. 25(10), pp. 1657–68.
Sha, Ji Cai (ed.) (1995), *The Position of Modern Chinese Women*, Beijing University Press, Beijing.
Shandong Provincial Government (2000), *Fee Schedule for Hospitals: The Third Version*, Jinan, Shandong.
Solinger, D. (1999), *Contesting Citizenship in Urban China: Peasant Migrants, the State and the Logic of the Market*, University of California Press, Berkeley.
Song, S. and Zhang, K. (2002), 'Urbanisation and City Size Distribution in China', *Urban Studies*, Vol. 39(12), pp. 2317–27.
Standing, H. (2001), 'A Framework for Incorporating Gender and Age into Social Policy Analysis in Urban China', unpublished paper available from the author at the Institute of Development Studies, Brighton, H.Standing@ids.ac.uk.
State Council (1996), *Improving Health Financial Policy*, China Economics Press, Beijing.
State Council (1998), *The Decision on Establishing Basic Health Insurance System for Urban Employees*, Beijing.
State Council (2000), *Guidelines for Urban Health and Medicine System Reform*, China Economics Press, Beijing.
Stockman, N. (1994), 'Gender Inequality and Social Structure in Urban China' *Sociology*, Vol. 28(3), pp. 759–77.
Strauss, A.L. (1987), *Qualitative Analysis for Social Scientists*, Cambridge University Press, Cambridge.
Sun, F. (1998), 'Ageing of the Population in China:Trends and Implications', *Asia-Pacific Population Journal*, Vol. 13(4), pp. 75–92.
Tang, J., Cook, S., Wang, L. and Ren, Z. (2000), 'Chengshi fupin wenti yu zuidi shenghuo baozhang zhidu yanjiu baogao', report prepared for workshop on urban poverty, Beijing, March 2000.
Tang, S., Lu, Y., Chen, J. and Bloom, G. (2001), 'How Did Enterprises Provide Health Care for Their Employees Under the Market Economy?' *Chinese Health Resource*, Vol. 4(5), pp. 198–200.
Tang, S.L., Tolhurst, R., Wang, Y. and Gao, J. (2001), 'Inequality in Access to Inpatient Services among Children in China: Analysis from a Gender Perspective', unpublished paper.
Tian, A.P., Lu, S.F. and Qu, L. (1999), 'The Situation of Reproductive Health Care Need and Provision for the Floating Population in Chengdu City', *Journal of Chinese Family Planning*, Vol. 7(5), Vol. 211–13.
Tu, F., Tokunaga, S., Deng, Z. and Nobutomo, K. (2002), 'Analysis of Hospital Charges For Cerebral Infarction Stroke Inpatients in Beijing, People's Republic of China', *Health Policy*, Vol. 59, pp. 243–56.
UNDP (United Nations Development Programme) (1999), *China Human Development Report – Economic Transition and Role of State*, China Finance and Economics Press, Beijing.
UNDP and ILO (2000), *Policies for Poverty Reduction in China*, United Nations Development Programme and International Labour Organization.
Wang, F. (1998), 'Chinese Health Insurance Reform: The Social Pooling Fund and Individual Account', *Chinese Journal of Health Economics*, Vol. 10, pp. 1–43.
Wang, F. and Zuo, X. (1999), 'Inside China's Cities: Institutional Barriers and Opportunities for Urban Migrants', *American Economic Review*, Vol. 89(2), pp. 276–80.

Wang, Kaiyu (1999), 'Analysis of Drug Expenses', *Chinese Hospital Management*, Vol. 3, pp. 18–19.

Wang, X. (2001), 'China's Pension System Reform and Capital Market Development,' presented to the International Conference on China and the WTO: the Financial Challenge, Kennedy School, Harvard University, 11–13 September 2001.

Wang, Y. and Wang, J. (1999), 'Zhenjiang Health Insurance Reform', *Chinese Journal of Health Service Administration*, Vol. 12, pp. 629–30.

Wang, Y.L., Ma, D.G. and Fang, J. (2000), 'The Immunization Issues Caused by Immigrant Population and the Corresponding Solution in Xiaoshan', *Chinese Rural Health Services Administration*, Vol. 20(3), pp. 41–2.

Wang, Y.P. (2001), 'Prospects and Problems of Urban Housing Reform', paper presented to Workshop on Social Policy Reform in Socialist Market China, Oxford, October 2001.

West, L. (1999), 'Pension Reform in China: Preparing for the Future', *Journal of Development Studies*, Vol. 35(3), pp. 153–83.

WHO (World Health Organization) (2003), 'SARS and Public Health Reform', draft white paper for the Government of China, Beijing.

Whyte, M.K. (1984), 'Sexual Inequality Under Socialism: The Chinese Case in Perspective' in J.L. Watson (ed.), *Class and Social Stratification in Post-Revolution China*, Cambridge University Press, Cambridge.

Wiley M.M. (1992), 'Hospital Financing Reform and Case-mix Measurement: An International Review', *Health Care Financing Review*, Vol. 13, pp. 119–33.

Williams, A. (1991), '"Need" – an Economic Exegesis', in A. Culyer (ed.), *The Economics of Health*, Vol. 1, Edward Elgar, Aldershot.

Wong, Chack-kie (1999), 'Reforming China's State Socialist Workfare System: A Cautionary and Incremental Approach', *Issues and Studies*, Vol. 35(5), pp. 169–94.

Wong, L. (1998), *Marginalization and Social Welfare in China*, Routlege, London.

World Bank (1996), *China: Issues and Options in Health Financing*, Report No. 15278-CHA, World Bank, Washington.

World Bank (1997), *China 2020 Issues and Options: Financing Health Care*, World Bank, Washington.

World Bank (2002), *China National Development and Sub-National Finance: A Review of Provincial Expenditures*, Report No. 22951-CHA, World Bank, Washington.

Wu, Ming (2002), 'Health Expenditure Control and Its Policies', unpublished report, Department of Health Policy and Management, School of Public Health, Beijing University.

Wu, Y., Xin, Y., Li, P. *et al.* (1999), 'The Problems and Support in Health Care Policy for Vulnerable Groups in Urban Communities', *Chinese Journal of Hospital Administration*, Vol. 15(8), pp. 466–7.

Wu, Y.S. (2003), 'A Survey on Pension System in Jilin and Helongjiang Provinces', *China Socail Welfare*, Vol. 6, pp. 45–8.

Xiang, X. and Shi, Y. (1997), 'Poverty to Diseases, Diseases Leading Back to Poverty', *Health Administration College Transaction*, Vol. 16(4), p. 238.

Xiao, X. (1999), 'Investigation on Child Health Care for Floating People', *Chinese Maternal and Child Health Care*, Vol. 14(12), pp. 761–2.

Xiong, Y. (1999), 'Social Policy for the Elderly in the Context of Ageing in China: Issues and Challenges of Social Work Education', *International Journal of Welfare for the Aged*, Vol.1, pp. 107–22.

Xu, F. (1998), 'Expenditure Under Labour Insurance Medical Service Scheme', *China Social Insurance*, No. 10, pp. 19–20.

Xu, K. *et al.* (1996), 'Economic Situation and Medical Expenditure of the Elderly in Shanghai', *Chinese Health Management*, Vol. 3, pp. 154–6.

Xu, K. *et al.* (1999), 'The Necessity of Medicaid for Poor People in Urban Area', *Chinese Health Policy*, Vol. 3, pp. 14–15.

Xu, K., Gong, X.G., Ying, X.H. *et al.* (1999), 'Theoretical Discussion on Medical Relief to Urban Poor Population', *Chinese Health Economics*, Vol. 18(1), pp. 19–21.

Xu, Lingzhu (2001), *Impacts of Hospital Financial Reform on Use of Health Resources. Technical Report*, Shandong University and University of New South Wales, Jinan.

Xue, M., Mao, J. and Chen, Y. (1999), 'Hospital Bed Occupancy Analysis: 1988–1997', *Chinese Hospital Management*, Vol. 19(3), pp. 31–3.

Yang, Feiqong (1998), 'Expenditure Under Labour Insurance Medical Service Scheme', *China Social Insurance*, pp. 19–20.

Yang, Huayou (1997), 'Effectiveness, Problems, and Policy Options in Reforming Urban Health Insurance Scheme in Jiujiang, *Chinese Health Economics*, Vol. 1(16), pp. 27–8.

Yang, Y. (1999), 'Challenge and Consideration to Population's Ageing', *Chinese Health Service Management*, Vol. 18(8), pp. 425–7.

Yip, W. and Eggleston, K. (2001), 'Provider Payment Reform in China: The Case of Hospital Reimbursement in Hainan Province', *Health Economics*, Vol. 10, pp. 325–39.

Yu, W. and Ren, M. (1998), 'The Conflicts of Social Ideals and Actual Interests – The Contradictions and Problems Existed in the Reform of Social Medical Insurance in the Towns of China', *Chinese Health Economics*, Vol. 17(9), pp. 5–8.

Yun, P. and Wang, W. (1990), *Zhongguo caishui gongzi baoxian fuli da quan* [Tax, Salary, Insurance and Welfare in China], Liao Ning People's Press, Shenyang.

Zhan, S., Sun, Z. and Blas, E. (2002), 'Economic Transitions and Maternal Health Care for Internal Migrants in Shanghai, China' *Health Policy and Planning*, Vol. 17 (Suppl. 1), pp. 47–55.

Zhan, Shaokang *et al.* (2000), 'Maternal Care for Internal Migrants in Shanghai', presented to the Conference on Rural Health Reform and Development in China, Beijing, November 2000.

Zhang, K., Ren, G.J. and Jiang, X.Y. (1999), 'Investigation on Emotional Status of Laid-off Workers', *Chinese Journal of Psychological Health*, Vol. 13(1), p. 34.

Zhang, L. (2002), 'Reform of the Household Registration (Hukou) System and Rural-Urban Migration in China: The Challenges Ahead', *Current Politics and Economics of China*, Vol. 3(3), pp. 481–509.

Zhang, L. *et al.* (1998), 'Analysis on Family Economic Risk for Diseases', *Chinese Rural Health Management*, Vol. 18(2), pp. 8–9.

Zhang, L.M. (1994), *Research on Women's Societal Position in Shanghai*, China Women's Press, Beijing.

Zhang, S., Cheng, C.Q., Liu, C. *et al.* (1999), 'Negative Psychological Behaviour, Its Cause and Possible Responses', *International Journal of Chinese Psychological and Physiological Medicine*, Vol. 1(4), p. 245.

Zhang, Wanli (2002), 'Twenty Years of Research on Stratified Social Structure in Contemporary China', *Social Sciences in China*, Vol. 23(1), pp. 48–58.

Zhang, X. *et al.* (1997), 'The Present State and Countermeasures of the Health Services to the Aged Inhabitants in Lanzhou Region', *Modern Preventive Medicine*, Vol. 24(4), pp. 410–12.

Zhang, Z. *et al.* (2000), 'Poverty Population and Health Services Utilization in the First World Bank Loan Counties', *Health Economic Research*, Vol. 18(11), pp. 25–32.

Zhao, H. *et al.* (2000), 'Investigation on Hospital Visits for Poverty Patients in Ningling Country', *Chinese Rural Health Management*, Vol. 20(9), pp. 27–9.

Zhao, Y. (1999), 'Estimation and Analysis of the National's Total Health Spending in 1996', *Chinese Health Economics*, Vol. 18(1), pp. 29–31.

Zhao, Zhuyan (1998), 'Improving Efficiency of Hospital Service Provision Through Reforming Health Care System', *Chinese Health Economics*, Vol. 17(5), pp. 8–9.

Zheng, Guoqiang (1996), 'Review of Labour Health Insurance Reform', *Chinese Hospital Management*, Vol. 12(10), pp. 598–600.

Zhong, H. *et al.* (1998), 'A Survey of Elder People's Quality of Life in Guanzhou City', *Chinese Journal of Nursing*, Vol. 33(6), p. 314.

Zhou, L.P. and Wang, R. Z. (1998), 'Analysis of Health Need and Utilisation of Elderly Population in Hangzhou City', *Journal of Zhejiang Medical University*, Vol. 27(2), pp. 84–7.

Zibo Bureau of Statistics (2000), *Zibo Statistical Yearbook*, Zibo.

Zibo Bureau of Statistics (2001), *Zibo Statistical Yearbook*, Zibo.

Zwanziger, J. and Melnick, G. (1988), 'The Effects of Hospital Competition and the Medicare PPOs Programme on Hospital Cost Behavior in California', *Journal of Health Economics*, Vol. 7, pp. 301–320.

Index

Milton Keynes UK
Ingram Content Group UK Ltd.
UKHW031130141024
449569UK00006B/294

9 780754 639664